How to Get the Most
Doctor

How to Get the Most from Your Doctor

Dr Jonathan Douglas

BLOOMSBURY

The examples given in this book are all taken from real cases and situations. Specifics have been changed to ensure that patients' confidentiality is protected.

First published as *How to Treat Your Doctor*.

This paperback edition first published 1993 by Bloomsbury Publishing Limited, 2 Soho Square, London W1V 5DE

Copyright © 1992 by Dr Jonathan Douglas

A CIP record for this book is available from the British Library

ISBN 0 7475 1292 2

10 9 8 7 6 5 4 3 2 1

Designed by Geoff Green
Typeset by Cambridge Composing (UK) Ltd
Printed by Cox & Wyman Ltd, Reading

For Jenny

Contents

Introduction

This book is about patients and doctors: their problems, their strengths, their weaknesses, and, particularly, the difficulties they have together.

The main focus is the consultation when patients and doctors talk and listen to one another. About 260 million consultations with family doctors took place in the UK last year. Most of these were not just about an 'illness' but a reflection of what modern life does to our minds and bodies. Figures show that on average women consult their doctors six times a year and men three times. Furthermore, the doctor is more likely to be consulted if his patient is unemployed, elderly or socially disadvantaged.

Getting the best out of these consultations is important: important for the patients so that problems are aired and illnesses attended to; important for the doctors so that they feel they are valued and that they are working effectively; important for society because of the doctors' pastoral role and the health of the nation.

For most of us illness is frightening, and we want to be treated quickly, continuously and correctly. At the heart of this experience should be a family doctor you can trust. The trust still seems to be there as a greater number of patients visit a doctor each year.

Doctors are spending more time with each patient and are issuing fewer prescriptions. However, the cost of these prescriptions is still rising and the financial pressure grows. What will the future hold? Some recent proposed financial changes for family doctors may prove to be an effective method of controlling spiralling costs. It may also prove to be a serious threat to the patient–doctor relationship.

In this book I hope to show just how special the patient–doctor relationship is and how important it is to fight for it.

Jonathan Douglas

1 First Meeting

The Practice 'Face'

Each medical practice has its own personality, beliefs, politics, style and behaviour. In most other social organizations there is a familiar structure. In schools there are head teachers and governors. In places of worship there are pastors and holy-days. In medical practices, however, there are few recognizable patterns or structures. There may be a reception desk or receptionists, but equally there may not; there is a nurse, sometimes, and a social worker, rarely. There are no set hours for opening and closing and appointments may or may not be made.

Many see this variation as the essential strength of general practice but the patient may feel lost and confused and frustrated. Patients passing from their old to their new general practice may recognize few familiar patterns.

How then are they to make best use of the services and resources available? Part of the answer may just be that in time it becomes familiar. But this answer is bad for patients and bad for general practice. It means there are a number of patients drifting around unable to make proper use of services and resources and unable to get the help they need when they need it. Today's patient usually wants a personalized welcome and service, up-to-date, informed, courteous staff and a range of services. Partly to satisfy the latter, a trend has developed over the years to group practices, but this also allows doctors the stimulation of working in groups and the benefits it brings to organization of work and leisure time.

Another answer is for it to be the expectation of every patient to be able to understand the personality, beliefs, politics, style and behaviour of the practice. The practice may already print an informal booklet which explains some of these issues. It will usually display opening hours, names of personnel, services, on-call and emergency arrangements. There may also be hints towards personality, politics and style in its presentation and content. However, the patient may still feel 'outside' the real character of the practice. He or she may get closer following a chat with the receptionist at registration or even closer following the first meeting with nurse or doctor. It is my belief that effective doctoring can only begin when there is mutual understanding between patient and the personnel of the practice. Getting that mutual understanding should be a priority for practice and patients.

In the sections which follow, these issues are explored in further depth. Firstly in understanding the system – the receptionists, the appointments, the on-call and emergency cover, and secondly in understanding one another – patients and professionals.

First Meeting Checklist

Questions for the Doctor
1   Does he/she have any particular interest or belief that has a bearing on my care? What is the ethos of the practice?
    For example:
    Dedicated to prevention: non-smoking groups; encouragement to self-help ideas such as yoga; medication counselling, rather than prescribing pills.
    Christian or other religious belief: referral for termination of pregnancy a difficulty?
    Strict financial control: some drugs too expensive to prescribe?

2 Can the doctor work with *my* particular interests, belief
and ethos?
For example:
Alternative therapies: medicines, homeopathy, religious
belief
3 Is the doctor happy to continue the treatment
prescribed by previous doctors?
4 Is there a doctor in the practice who takes a particular
interest in my complaint/illness?

The Practice Reception and Receptionists

Let us start with an ideal, or is it a fantasy?

The practice reception is the practice 'face'. This face may be
open and welcoming. The reception staff may have been well
trained to value their skills in greeting and interviewing patients.
They may be aware of how frightening it is to feel ill and how
difficult it is for many patients to get to the surgery at all. They
are in tune with the 'patient' within themselves. They will often
be helping disabled people through doors, holding babies when
a parent is in with the doctor and lifting pushchairs down stairs.
They will have the experience to spot a crisis, will have learnt
how to defuse anger and in all this to protect confidentiality.
These receptionists try to balance the immediate needs of the
patients with the finite resources of practice consultation time.
In order to do the job well the receptionist needs to have a
mature and sensitive personality.

These remarkable people are likely to be supported by their
environment. There will be a warm welcoming atmosphere in
reception. This welcome may extend to flowers on the desk,
pleasant decor and thoughtful architecture. The reception area
will be open with patients at the same eye level as the receptionists. The contact will be free from screens or glass panels and
there will be an area set aside for confidential and sensitive
conversations. The reception area will have notices about practice organization and services to patients. These will be easy to

understand and in language free from jargon, and translated to reflect the cultural makeup of the practice profile. The practice leaflet will be offered to all patients and will give an idea of the attitudes and ethos of the practice.

Enough of fantasy; the reality is different. The patient will often find the reception area and staff who work there distant and bureaucratic. They may be physically separated from the care they want by closed doors with short surgery hours. Contact is via glass panels or screens through which they must shout their personal details. Receptionists on high stools peer down apparently in judgement of need. Hostile notices will remind the patient that home visits have to be in by 10 a.m. and that patients turning up late will not be seen. The reception area is often cramped and the waiting area restricted, with insufficient seats and little in the way of toys or magazines.

If the practice reception *is* the practice face and that face appears to frown then this is often because the doctors mean it so. Many believe that 'nannying' patients makes them dependent on the medical world and destroys self-reliance; if the surgery is too welcoming and the staff too understanding it will encourage the lonely and disadvantaged to tarry there. Many doctors believe that their practices should reflect the world outside, their practice area. Here being disorganized, emotionally frail or vulnerable carries disadvantage. Why should doctors put up with late-comers to appointments, people who can't even cope with making an appointment or those unable to state clearly and confidently to a receptionist the care they require? These doctors see it as government responsibility to provide a clear social policy to protect those in need and would be disturbed to think of themselves as a modern church providing an oasis of care for those fallen from the jetstream of modern success.

The patient at reception may, however, be feeling alienated — not by the practice policy but by more everyday human failure. It may be that the receptionists are hostile because they are expected to cope with an unrealistic number of tasks by a practice with poor management and low staff pay levels. They may include a member of the doctor's family who is fed up with patients seeming always to encroach on family life. These staff may be impossible to 'sack' without splitting the partnership. Reception unhappiness is often a reflection of a dispute between the doctors which has failed to be resolved.

The receptionist may 'protect' the doctor from 'difficult' patients and allow the doctor to be seen as the good guy or gal. The receptionist may also be hostile because the doctor lays down strict rules about organization which the staff dutifully follow, only to see the doctor himself ignoring those same rules when dealing with patients.

Sick doctors may rely on receptionists to cover for their illnesses or drug/drink dependency. The loyal receptionist, having watched the caring doctor fall apart, following a marital split or death in the family, may well take on tasks outside of her work. She may give medical advice over the phone, dress wounds and write prescriptions for the doctor to sign.

The reception may also be unhappy as the cramped working environment may reflect poor building design and insufficient funding by government to allow for a pleasant working environment.

So where does this leave the patient? If you are joining a practice what should you look for at reception and what should you want from the staff there? The following is a checklist of things to find out when joining a new practice.

Organization Checklist
1   Get practice leaflet – is there a clear list of services and personnel? There should be information about:
      Appointments system
      Saturday surgeries
      Urgent consultations
      Nurses
      Disabled patients
      Visits
      Clinics
      Repeat prescriptions
      Practice area
      How to get to the surgery

2　If unclear, ask about on-call arrangements when the practice is closed. Does the practice use a deputizing service and when does that come into operation?

3　How does the practice make appointments for the patient to be seen? Can an urgent problem really be seen quickly? Are children's illnesses given priority? Can you make a longer appointment with the doctor for difficult problems?

4　How personal is the service? Are patients encouraged to stay with one doctor? Can patients change to another doctor if they don't get on?

5　How are regular medicines dispensed or prescribed? Can you get a repeat prescription left out or returned in an sae?

Practice Checklist for Staff, Doctors and Patients

1　*Evidence that patients' comfort and welfare has been considered*
Chairs comfortable even if cramped; warm waiting area with thought given to children's play and adults' reading matter. Friendly staff. Space for confidential conversations; tissues for tears; privacy when undressing. Arrangements for nursing mothers, nappy changing. Special consideration given to seriously ill patients. Assistance for the disabled and thought given to those with English as a second language. A greeting from doctors, nurses and receptionist.

2　*Evidence that the practice is well organized*
Practice information leaflets available and relevant. Staff appear well trained. A variety of services to patients. Reception area, toilets, waiting area, all clean.

3　*Evidence of flexibility, change and initiative*
Longer appointments available for more serious issues; urgent appointments available. Willingness to treat those with differing views and attitudes. Telephone availability of doctors. Surgery hours to reflect differing

needs of the community. A sense that the staff and doctors could apologize for getting things wrong.

In summary, the evidence for a sick or healthy practice is there in the reception area. How are we, the patients, to trust our doctors if the surgery toilet is always filthy, if the receptionists are hostile, and nothing is done about it? How can our doctors organize our treatments if they can't organize a reception area to provide a sensitive service?

Understanding the System

Appointments

Every practice has its own system. Some will prefer the turn up and wait system based on the 'first come first served' principle. It has the great advantage that the patients know that they will be seen even if it means waiting. It has, however, many disadvantages. It can lead to large numbers queueing in bad weather waiting for the practice to open. The system favours those who are most able to get up early and those without other responsibilities or without disability. It is clearly difficult for the single parent, for those with a number of children, for the elderly, for the disabled and for those who are in paid work with a busy schedule of meetings and responsibilities. It is both good and bad for the doctors. Good in that on quiet days the workload is light and there is unexpected time for other activities, e.g. catching up on reading the literature (journals etc); bad in that on busy days there may be more patients to be seen than is really consistent with good patient care. There is also insufficient time for other duties such as home visiting. This stop–start system also means that planning is difficult both in terms of patient care and in terms of the doctors' personal lives.

At the other end of the scale is a rigid system of appointments. The patient may feel that he or she has 'to book to be ill' as by the time an appointment is available she is usually better or much worse. The system has advantages for the busy time slaves in the world, but may make ill patients wait too long.

It seems the answer is in the middle: on one hand surgeries can be booked well in advance and these are kept to time; on the other hand there are surgeries for the emergency or urgent cases. This middle option needs a careful understanding of the system by patients and staff. It may be that the urgent cases are dealt with by the practice partners in rotation, running a walk-in surgery. Alternatively, these patients may be seen before or after the booked surgery is held. Patients and staff will have to work hard to make this system work well: first, making sure that only urgent problems are dealt with in the urgent slots and on-going problems referred to the receptionists for appointments; second, making sure that patients finding that urgent slots are the quickest way into the service don't abuse the system by bringing any problem at these times, however trivial; finally, making sure that well-meaning and non-assertive patients don't hold on to urgent symptoms feeling guilty about taking an urgent appointment and preferring to wait until a booked appointment is available.

Education is the key, and practices make efforts to 'train' their patients to use the service provided. One practice has thought of an unusual system to improve waiting times and efficiency. It was decided to offer consultations of varying length: very short, medium or very long. The patient could then make an appointment for two minutes to get a document signed or certificate issued, or alternatively, for much longer if his or her partner had just died or a full length medical was required. Time-keeping by this method is shared, the patient taking some responsibility for ending the consultation on time so as not to disadvantage others. This sounds a nightmare to organize but has obvious advantages.

The practice leaflet may show you the times your doctor is available. It may also give details of emergency or urgent appointments. It would be even better if the receptionists had time to welcome every new patient and explain the system face to face. The patient in turn may want to pose situation questions to get a better grasp of how this practice organizes care:

My Jackie gets asthma. Sometimes I get sufficient warning but occasionally it's urgent. If I've had a bad night with her, can I always bring her in?

I don't finish work until 6 p.m.. Do you have late appointments?

Can I make a longer appointment to see the doctor about my mother. It's such a long story and I always feel rushed.

Questions such as these may expose the limits and weaknesses in a particular system. No practice can offer a system that is totally suitable and convenient for doctors and patients.

In my own practice we attempt to give time and space to patients with serious problems. We recognize that if a problem is explored in detail initially then further appointments may not be necessary. This, however, can cause chaos to appointments and extend other patients' waiting time. Other practices may run to time but can leave the patient and doctor feeling that a problem has been shelved or only partially sorted out.

On Call

From the patients' point of view, an 'out of hours call' is usually a crisis. Perhaps a screaming, hot child; severe pain or vomiting after dinner; or a sudden psychiatric crisis. At these times patients want a quick, informed service that does not involve unnecessary telephone calls or lengthy negotiation with go-betweens.

Family doctors are responsible for the medical needs of their patients 24 hours a day. This requirement is written in their Terms and Conditions of Service. It is understood that some doctors will make arrangements to share this responsibility with partners, or, in a small practice, with a neighbouring practice of a similar size. Some single-handed family doctors will cover their patients 24 hours a day, only getting a paid replacement (a locum) at times of holidays and special occasions. In inner city and other highly populated areas, commercial companies employing doctors provide night-time cover (deputizing service) for a large number of doctors. The local management structure for GPs ensures that this service is not used to excess and to the detriment of continuous medical care of patients.

Deputizing service

For the patient joining a new practice it is important to understand which system is used and when – for instance, if the practice employs the deputizing service to cover night calls, and just when the practice switches over to this service. For patients this information is particularly useful. It may be that they are caring for a sick child or elderly relative and have been in touch with the practice during the day. If the partners of the practice are available until 11 p.m. then advice is likely to be consistent and relevant to that particular practice. The doctors will know precisely the arrangements for care the following day and there will be continuity of care.

If, however, the patient rings for advice at 11.05 p.m. the call will be referred to the commercial deputizing agency who will provide an emergency service, including home visiting, but they will not know the detailed practice arrangements. It may be that rather than wait until morning for a review, the patient will be referred to hospital at an earlier stage. This defensive medicine is safe, particularly as the visiting doctor has to make the clinical judgements without the family and past medical knowledge available to the family doctors. However, it is not necessarily the most efficient use of resources.

Ideally, the family doctor is in the best position to make the correct judgement. However, the demands on his or her time by a full list of patients often means that that judgement can be impaired by tiredness. Getting the balance right is difficult.

On one side there is the belief that the family doctor's life is a vocation and the patients are all-important. The hardships of overtiredness and unsocial hours come with the job and are to be accepted. On the other side is the belief that a rested doctor will provide a better opinion under stress. Doctors too need stable home lives in order to give balanced judgements. The job is more a job than a lifelong vocation. In teaching young family doctors, I sense a move to the second description. They are less likely than the generation before them to accept the long hours and antisocial working environments. They are more aware of the need to care for themselves if they are to care for others. This change has implications for the future.

Emergency

What is an emergency? There are some we can all agree on: a heart attack, a stroke, a suicide attempt, an asthma attack. But what about the bad headache, the tummy pain, or a heavy period or even the fifteen-year-old with a request for the morning-after-pill? Each patient has their own view of when to call the doctor:

> I remember one night being called to an elderly lady who couldn't be woken from sleep. Her husband had got her to sit in the chair after dinner as washing up had brought on chest pain. Despite her pain, her breathlessness and her lips turning blue, he wouldn't call the doctor. He had been brought up to call the doctor only if someone was dangerously ill and, to his mind, his wife was just having a 'turn'. When I arrived she had clearly been dead for some time. I wondered just how fierce these parents were who taught their son about these rules and just what sort of doctors demanded such protection. I had a picture of top-hatted, Edwardian medical men arriving by horse carrying the fear and respect of the community. How would these doctors have treated another elderly woman who, having patiently listened to the recorded message '. . . in absolute medical emergency please ring . . .' had indeed rung at 3 a.m. to say, 'Is that the doctor? Oh good. I just wanted to know you were there.'

What guidance is there for today's patients about when to call the doctor? Where does the advice come from now that the extended family network is less common? Grandparents seem less in evidence to reassure parents about common illnesses. Perhaps modern patients are right to question what is safe and what is not when so much in our environment is under threat.

How can we feel reassured about illnesses when things we used to be sure of have let us down – the climate, the safety of tap water, eggs, additives and pesticides in food . . .?

Looking back over last year's diary of emergency calls, there seems to be no pattern. There *is* a kaleidoscope of suffering, fear, anxiety, sadness and, of course, occasional joy. It is easy to remember some emergencies: the call from an elderly man who was vomiting blood and who collapsed while on the phone, then the mad rush to get to his house and break the door down to get him to hospital; or the visit to the man with an epileptic fit who was carried from the third floor down steep stairs on a stretcher to an ambulance; or even the unexpected birth in the front hall next to the suitcase packed ready for hospital. . . . Then there is the truly unexpected: the visit to a medical family for a son with flu and a few spots. I had thought this was just a mild illness and more evidence of how difficult it is for the parent to judge when medically qualified herself. Instead here was a dangerously ill boy suffering with the signs of a rare septicaemia from which he was lucky to survive. In the same week I was called by a local policeman who had found an isolated elderly man dead at home. He had fallen awkwardly with his head under a chest of drawers and had suffered extensive head injuries before he died. The policeman had felt his limbs and he was icy cold. As we pulled him out we both jumped as he groaned loudly – a modern-day Lazarus! And a few weeks later I was called to a local grocery store. The owner was disturbed by the person standing in his shop. She had recently been discharged from mental hospital nearby. She had crossed a busy street in mid-afternoon stark naked and was in the process of picking her own fruit and vegetables.

These examples stay in the memory as would rare birds to bird-watchers. It is easy to forget the hundreds of 'sparrows and starlings' which are just as important: the first high fever in the first-born child; the angry immobility of a slipped disc in a young man; the pain and sadness of miscarriage as a couple cradle the recently expelled fetus; the severity of influenza; the fearful noise of a crouping child; the pain of earache in children; the relief as a catheter is passed into the bladder of one who can't 'go'; the breathless exhaustion of asthma; the perplexity of the confused, and the peace in the dead.

Looking again at this year's emergency calls, it now seems clear that patient and doctor knowing each other is the best basis for judgements. If the patient has been through a number of contacts or illnesses with his doctor and built up trust, then acceptance of reassurance, even without being seen, is often enough. Similarly, if the doctor knows his patient then he can fill in those pieces of the jigsaw which are not there at the time of the emergency call. This will mean some patients will get urgent visits with little discussion and others will get advice on the telephone prior to any visit later in the day.

What to do in an emergency

When patients first join their new practice they should of course receive some information about how to contact a doctor in the event of an emergency. They should also consider it part of their health care to understand the attitudes about emergencies in the practice. If they suffer with a longstanding medical complaint they would need to understand at what point help should be sought and where to get such advice.

On Call/Emergency Checklist

1 Find out and write down your family doctor's telephone number (day-time, out-of-hours and emergency). Post these numbers somewhere obvious where babysitters, grandparents, partially sighted people can see them.

2 Discuss on-call and emergency arrangements with your doctor, especially if you or dependants have a serious or unpredictable illness, e.g. asthma.

3 Know the practice arrangements for emergency cover, e.g. when and to whom they hand over emergency cover.

4 Ask about any possible time delay and any actions to be taken when waiting.

5 *Remember:* ambulance 999; practise dialling *now* (leave receiver down) and practise dialling with your eyes closed!

Understanding Each Other

First Meeting – Negotiating a Working Relationship

What does it feel like to be a new patient joining an unfamiliar practice? I think that sometimes it must feel like a passenger catching a train just as it is leaving the station. The passenger, like the patient, may be unsure that this is the right train going in the right direction. Furthermore, the passenger has no idea if the driver is competent. Of course, passengers can leave the train at the next station as patients can leave doctors. But what if this is the only train and the doctor the only one for miles?

In an ideal world there would be time to sit down and look at the practice and the staff who work there. The practice too would have a chance to meet you and see just what sort of 'passenger' you are. It is, however, more common for patients to find a doctor when they are ill and to make that choice when they are anxious or unwell. Often that meeting is pressed for time and the idea of 'negotiating a working relationship' seems unrealistic.

No matter whether this first meeting is when the patient is ill or whether the patient or doctor has requested a meeting on joining the practice, it is a golden opportunity. The opportunity to set the tone for the future: to show each other's values and beliefs. The opportunity also to mark out 'boundaries' and 'who's in charge' and to explore anger, embarrassment, fear and language (see Chapter 2). Like most first meetings, immediate impressions mean a lot. Getting it right straight away is not essential (see Chapter 3), but despite the many difficulties likely to be present in such a first meeting, there are opportunities to get on the right track.

It might go like this:

Mr Stevens isn't it? Hello, I'm Doctor Perkins; have a seat; now how can I help you?

How might the new patient feel and how will the patient behave? The patient has been briefly welcomed and introduced. The doctor appears business-like and is keen to get on with the problem.

It might also go like this:

> Hello Mr Stevens. I'm Doctor Perkins; nice to meet you; please sit down. Before you tell me what's wrong, can I ask you to give some information about yourself, your background, health and family?

How does the patient feel now? Is this a better start? Will it necessarily lead to a better working relationship?

If there is pressure of time does this sound better:

> Mr Stevens isn't it? Hello, I'm Doctor Perkins; have a seat. As you can see, it's very busy out there today. Do you mind if we only talk about your present complaint and meet up another time to get to know each other better?

Is this welcome a better start? Does the patient feel more understood and valued by the last example than by the first? Even from just one brief conversation, there can be infinite impressions made.

So much for the doctor's opening lines; what about the patient's?

> Hello Doc, nice to meet you. I've just moved into the area. You won't be seeing much of me, I didn't worry my old doc much. All I need is a repeat prescription for my sleeping pills.

What will the doctor feel and how will he or she behave with this opening 'ticket'? The doctor might feel that the patient is overfamiliar, controlling and presumptuous. But he might also feel that the patient is considerate and realistic. This impression might produce the following reply:

> I'm afraid you're going to find things different here – we don't issue repeat prescriptions for sleeping tablets.

or

> Why don't you sit down and tell me about yourself before talking
> about sleeping tablets?

or even

> I feel you are trying to tempt me into giving you your sleeping
> tablets by promising me a quiet life if I do.

The issues of 'who's in charge', expressing anger, and establishing boundaries (more on these later) are already on view. Here's another example:

> Hello, it is nice to meet you Dr Perkins. What a pleasant surgery.
> My old doctor worked in a dreadful place. Now that I'm here I
> would really like a complete check-up. I've heard we should all
> have a thorough medical yearly and an ovary scan every three
> years. Oh, by the way, I usually have my cholesterol checked
> every few months.

Some doctors might think 'Ah, a patient who is interested and involved in prevention and taking responsibility for her health.' Other doctors might think 'Who does this woman think she is? This is the Health Service! If I did yearly medicals on everyone it would mean 60 medicals a week, and what about the sick and needy?' Still others might think: 'I wonder what made this woman behave like this?'

But these are impressions, prejudices and attitudes; they are not facts. 'Tell me about yourself; tell me about your family/ past health/relationships/work/exercise/recreation,' this is more likely to reveal the facts.

Patients are usually remarkably open with their doctors. Discovering the serious illness as a child or the early death of a father can be crucial, just as crucial as the family history of diabetes or high blood pressure. What is the patients' work and how do they feel about it? What relationships have they got and who is in the family?

Many practices have a practice card to prompt them to record this information. It might look like this:

FEMALE 3 YEARLY CHECK

Date	B.P.	Weight	Height	Urine	Cervical Smear

Tetanus:-

Rubella: Vaccination: Immune Status:

Obstetric History: Blood Group: Hysterectomy

Date   Contraception:

FP1001
CLAIM

Date   D.O.B.   FEMALE

SURNAME   Forenames

Address

Tel Home:-   Work:-

Occupation

Smoking   Alcohol

Exercise

D.M.   HT/♡   THY.   GLAUC

Relationship

Date   Past Medical History   Allergies

See Over

Date 1.2.91 D.O.B. 28.2.40 FEMALE

SURNAME SMITH Forenames Evelyn, M.

Address 10 Pages Hill
ThisHeborough HANTS

Tel Home: 0723 64372 Work: 0723 465 63

Occupation F.E. Teacher Computers

Smoking Nil Alcohol 10 units/wk

Exercise Yoga 2xs wk

D.M. ✓ HT ⊙ Bronchy THY. ✓ GLAUC ✓

Relationship

Lung Cancer
† @ 56   72 well
○   ○

John □ ○ Jam
50   48
Obese OK
Smokes
⊙ Dis.

○ Joan   □ □ Terry Obese   □ Frank
  1971   1974   51
              Smokes   Obese

Date	Past Medical History	Allergies PENICILLIN
1984	VV's Done	
1989	D&C for Menorrhagia	

See Over

FEMALE 3 YEARLY CHECK

Date	B.P.	Weight	Height	Urine	Cervical Smear
7.4.86	120/70	64.4	167	NAD	1985 OK
6.5.89	130/90	66.0	167	NAD	1988 OK

Tetanus:- 1975 ✓ 1985 ✓

Rubella: Vaccination: Immune Status: 1971

Blood Group O+   Hysterectomy

Obstetric History: 1971 Forceps delivery, Normal Preg/Pun
1974 Normal Vaginal Delivery's Preg.

Contraception:

Date
1974
↓
Sheath

FP1001
CLAIM

At a glance the family structure is visible. Supposing Evelyn Smith came to her doctor with insomnia and mentioned being worried about her 17-year-old son: he has become increasingly rude and aggressive, and she mentions that 'it's so much easier with my students at work'. The profile card would remind the doctor that Evelyn teaches computing at a Further Education college. But when she goes on to mention that Terry has started smoking the doctor can understand Evelyn's particular anxiety as she has a brother with heart disease and a father who died of lung cancer. The easy access to this sort of information can make the difference in whether the patient feels understood or not.

The patient is often asked to fill in a questionnaire on joining the practice and this information may then be transposed onto the card. Asking for this detailed information, particularly if followed up with a meeting with doctor or nurse, can give the patient a sense of being welcomed and valued. The questionnaires have to be worded carefully and reassurance given as to the level of confidentiality in the surgery. The reverse of the card shows details concerning past health and a reminder of checks to come in the future.

These early visits to the practice can give the doctors and nurses a clear picture of their patient, but what of the patient's view? After all, doctors are on familiar ground in their own space, surrounded by a range of social and professional supports. The name on the door, the equipment and uniform all announce status. How then can patients be assertive in these circumstances?

How often do doctors hear:

Now that you've asked me a bit about myself, can I check a few points about you and the practice?

Do you feel that someone my age should have check-ups?

Can I always see you in the surgery?

If we don't get on, can I see your partner?

What's your attitude to alternative medicines? Will you treat
Jehovah's Witnesses?

It seems reasonable to expect and encourage such questions.
Establishing where both parties stand bodes well for the future
and may prevent difficulties (see Chapter 2).

But it is, of course, an unequal relationship. It is unreasonable
for the patient to expect to know details of the doctor's personal
and private life. This would interfere with the objective judgements that doctors and patients make. If, however, the patient
wanted to know the doctor's stance on abortion, private practice, or confidentiality of consultations with under-18s, then
these seem questions that should be answered.

Trust

I work down the hill from an old village which is surrounded
and invaded by inner city life. The trunk roads carry the city
work force and heavy goods vehicles past dusty properties full
of bedsits. Large council high-rises are hidden behind leafy rows
of owner-occupied properties.

Working in a village means that news travels fast. The
reputation of the practice will be known and passed from lip to
lip; its faults and strengths dissected. If the practice is thought
generally to provide a safe, caring service to the community,
then a reserve of trust is established. This reserve will be called
upon when things go wrong, such as a missed appendix or the
broken answerphone. How much patients and doctors depend
on this reserve can be seen in everyday practice. If in the future
the reserve of trust should be threatened by political change,
then the results will be far reaching (see Chapter 4).

In the practice I work in nearly 15 per cent of patients move
each year. This will mean a new patient joining my list and an
old patient leaving every day. One patient who recently left had
visited the practice 325 times over the last 31 years. She had
certainly trusted us with her health, or rather, ill health.
Unfortunately, she had been unable to trust herself to remain
well unless she visited the doctor frequently.

New patients arrive in the surgery and begin the process of registration and introduction to the practice. They may have come to register now, because they are feeling unwell. As they come for their first consultation I am struck by the level of trust already established. Most patients, after a brief introduction, are prepared to sit down and talk about their lives to this total stranger. This trust may have come from village talk. It may also be from fond memories of *Dr Finlay's Casebook* or *Dr Kildare*. It may in part be from the warm welcome of receptionists or the past experience with a previous doctor. It also may be present because of those vulnerable feelings when we are ill. We may hope that this stranger, the doctor, will take control – as a parent might – to make us feel better. I was reminded of these feelings when in hospital recently; I had implicit faith in the staff nurse and hung on her every word.

A reserve of trust is also given by society. Doctors are normally portrayed as responsible and well trained. The doctors' parent organization, the General Medical Council, is aware just how much doctors are trusted. They consider breaches of this trust, such as drunkenness or sexual harassment of patients, to be the most serious misdemeanours. These offences are given wide publicity to doctors to remind them of the severe penalties imposed.

This general trust is of course naïve. It has not been earned by the individual doctor and can cause difficulties in the patient–doctor relationship. The over-trusted doctor can start to make decisions in the patient's 'best interests' without being in real touch with the patient. Fortunately, there are sufficient numbers of patients who keep us nearer reality. To them, Dr Kildare is a smarmy egomaniac and their last family doctor a disaster. Real trust is not a gift from soap operas, it is a contract. This contract will need frequent revision as the relationship changes and matures. Here follow some examples.

Mr Patel arrived as a new patient. He worked as an accountant. He had registered that day because of a return of his sinus infection. He explained that his previous doctor had advised him to get antibiotics early on in the infection to prevent it getting established. I carefully examined him and found that despite his rather nasal voice he had no evidence of sinusitis. It was no more than a bit of catarrh. I explained my usual 'spiel' of how we must avoid antibiotics if possible. I could feel that he wanted to agree with me but experience had taught him differently. I thought I would need to work even harder to get him to see my point of view. I invited him to come back three days later if he felt he was worse. At the reception desk he booked the appointment. I expected he would ring to cancel it. Three days later he arrived with a fever and tender sinuses; he had been right. I gave him the antibiotics. As time has passed and he has had two further episodes, I began to see his past GP's point of view. I asked him to come in to discuss it. We agreed that he was the best person to judge when the attack was coming. He should therefore hold a supply of the antibiotics to take at the 'correct' time for him. He was pleased to receive this trust and told me how much this would help him. He would no longer need to be ringing up trying to get appointments and face explaining the story each time. On my part, I suggested some other ways that an attack could be averted. He was prepared to try a particular nasal spray at the first sign of congestion. He has found that this in fact does put off more than half of his sinusitis attacks and has decided to carry the spray with him.

This is a simple example of trust building in a doctor–patient relationship. We will face future problems with some mutual trust in the 'bank'. Sometimes the issues of trust are more complicated.

I was the new partner, just arrived. Each surgery was a challenge as I did not know the local services or the hospital doctors, let alone my partners and my patients! Each patient seemed to have come to see the new doctor and negotiate their own special relationship. An Australian woman in her thirties came in and announced she was pregnant. She was pleased but frightened. Her last pregnancy had been normal but after the baby was born she had become severely depressed and needed admission to mental hospital. She had made a full recovery but remembered her suicidal thoughts with a shudder. She explained how she was sure this wouldn't happen again if only she could avoid going to the hospital. She hated the antenatal clinic, the postnatal wards and distrusted the obstetric staff generally. She was determined to have a home birth. She had read about other women's experiences and felt sure it would be all right this time. There was no medical reason why she should not proceed, and I felt it was only right to support her decision. I felt that to question her further about her past experience and her real anxieties now would be to undermine her confidence. I felt that she would need to trust herself, her doctor and her midwife completely for her to stand the best chance of avoiding a further breakdown. The pregnancy progressed, she stayed optimistic throughout.

It was my first home birth to attend with the job, and I hid my anxieties. I felt I could not talk about the potential problems as I would reveal the patient's and my own anxiety. We travelled together on a 'fantasy voyage' not daring to look too carefully at the map.

The birth at home was a great success. Husband, wife, midwife and doctor toasted the new baby. There was an atmosphere of success and achievement that felt permanent. But it was not to be. When the baby was a week old, the depression returned suddenly. Martha was desperately ill and she and the new baby had to be admitted to hospital for their own safety.

Months later Martha came in and I asked her whether she wanted to talk about the whole experience now that she was well. She was furious with me. She had trusted me to such an extent that she believed I could protect her from this illness. She felt cheated and let down.

We discussed it further and I accepted the criticism. In supporting her decision I hoped to reinforce her self-belief. I wanted to trust her judgement and prove that my rather pessimistic training in psychiatry could be wrong. In fact, I allowed the patient to become dependent to support my own anxiety. She explained how she thought that a more thorough look at her fears and fantasies of illness would have provided better protection. She also thought it would have been better to remain neutral and open about the possible return of depression. In retrospect my failure to talk about it implied to her that she might appear too fragile to handle it. I talked about my need for this first home birth to go well and she had picked up on this.

Our honest discussion was healing and it has been possible to re-establish the contact on a more realistic footing.

Subsequently, she has had two more pregnancies and has prevented a further bout of depression by deciding to take medicines immediately after birth.

Risk-Taking

We all take risks every day: we might take the risk in jumping a red light or leaving off the seat belt; we measure up whether to travel by air or train; we lean a little too far on the ladder or unplug the kettle with damp hands.

We also take risks in relationships: physical risks such as not wearing a condom or the playful tap that's just too hard; and emotional risks, such as admitting we're frightened or jealous.

Patients and doctors often discuss risks: What are the risks of a particular treatment and what would be the risk if no treatment was taken? How can this patient be so worried about food additives and yet smoke 40 a day? Why does the vegetarian marathon runner never sit down and relax? How come my dad smoked, and drank like a fish and lived to 90?

We may all decide that despite the wisdom of low-risk living it is just too difficult to make a change. For instance, a policeman came in with another chest infection. 'I know it's the smoking,' he said, 'but there's no way I can stop at the moment.' I asked him what would need to change to make it possible for him to stop the cigarettes. 'A bloody miracle,' came the reply, 'that's what. You know what it's like down there – we're short-staffed and all leave's been cancelled. On top of that my John's gone and got a girl in trouble.'

The cigarettes seemed irrelevant when I listened to his list of troubles. But I was in for a surprise. I saw him a month or two later, he looked fitter and happier. He described how, shortly after our discussion, his brother had lost the circulation to a leg.

The artery was blocked and he needed an amputation. The surgeon explained it was going to be the other leg soon unless he stopped smoking. That was the miracle. Both brothers stopped smoking. The risk had seemed acceptable until it became more real. Catching that moment for change is one of the joys of family doctoring.

In one area of family medicine, risks should be encouraged. This is the area of the consultation. For this to happen a measure of trust needs to be established (see Chapter 1). As there is insufficient time for a complete and detailed analysis of mind and body, doctors and patients have to take short cuts: hunches have to be followed and gut feelings revealed. Both doctors and patients have to take the risk.

> When we called you the other night I got the feeling you thought we were wasting your time.

> You're talking to me as if you don't expect me to get better.

> When I hear you speak of your mother I sense a feeling of guilt.

> Please tell me if I'm wrong but I feel you distrust my judgement.

The statements based on received feelings cut through to the heart of a problem. If doctors can show that they are prepared to take a risk then it encourages the patient to do the same.

> Elizabeth, a nurse, consulted frequently. Initially it was for a flu-like illness and tiredness, but gradually the consultations moved on to discuss a number of gynaecological complaints. Her periods never seemed just right, one month too heavy and too long, the next too early and too light. She also complained of a vaginal discharge but there never seemed to be much evidence. I felt we were getting nowhere. I tried to explore her current relationship as a possible cause for her symptoms but drew a blank. One morning when another vaginal symptom presented, 'Elizabeth,' I ventured, 'I get the feeling that something awful has happened to you and your vagina.'

> She broke down in tears and spoke for the first time about her sexual abuse as a child. Her uncle 'looked after' her and her sister when their parents were away on short trips abroad. He

would visit her bedroom at night and in the darkness touch her vagina and encourage her to masturbate him. He told her that should she tell her parents he would explain he had noticed night-time noises and a tendency to touch herself whenever she could. This secret had remained locked away all this time and now was out in the open. Over the months she took the risk to talk to her boyfriend about it. She even talked to her sister who to her surprise had suffered in the same way. Eventually they confronted the parents and sought from them an apology for failing to protect their daughters.

The uncle could not be brought to trial as he had died some months before Elizabeth's symptoms began. Nevertheless, he was seen to be guilty as the parents remembered other evidence that should have alerted them when the girls were young.

Elizabeth took the risk initially by coming to the doctor. Listening to her and feeling that the problem didn't add up was the clue for the doctor to take a risk. In such a situation, if the doctor had got it wrong the patient would usually have accepted the doctor was trying to help. In fact, they then may be encouraged to try out a 'hunch' themselves to explain their symptoms.

Foibles

As trust develops between doctor and patient, each other's foibles can be revealed. These slight peculiarities are *tolerated* and can add colour and interest.

My trainer in general practice had noticed how patients with heart pain were worse when the cold east wind blew as they walked down to the surgery. He insisted that they should put newspaper inside their vests to protect the front of the chest. On cold days he would tap their shirts as they walked through the surgery door expecting to hear the crackle of protective newspaper. I would see them furtively removing it as they left the surgery; they knew that the man in there really cared for them and his foible was a minor irritation only.

One elderly man would always try to show me his army exercises before he left the surgery. In particular he would say, 'See doctor, I can still kick my own height?' He would then leap up and demonstrate. I thought I understood what he was really saying and now that he no longer can, his depression is that bit deeper.

A rather eccentric elderly lady with cats was in the surgery one day talking about her arthritis. As she talked on, I noticed it had started raining and storm clouds were gathering. She became restless, and let out with a blood curdling shriek as the first flash of lightning came down. With no regard to her arthritis she leapt up onto the examination couch and stood in the corner whimpering. She was truly afraid of lightning and had been caught out by the speed of the developing storm. The reception staff got her down and managed to calm her with tea and biscuits.

Another patient, troubled by her past, would come and talk about her parenting. She hoped she could avoid passing on problems to her own children and was seeking help with this. As she described her own childhood she would pick up paper clips from my desk and twist them into miniature sculptures of her pain and suffering. They were always left behind in the surgery.

These are but a few examples of foibles. My own are probably noticed by my patients but so far they have been too polite to mention them.

Culture and Belief

The patients' and doctors' beliefs will not usually become clear at the first meeting. However, cultural differences may be obvious from language, dress, race or behaviour. The Sikh doctor in his turban facing a leather-studded Hell's Angel may seem poles apart. Both may make assumptions about the other. But if they can hold off their prejudice and give each other a chance then something important may come of it. (Difficulties in these areas are explored in greater detail in Chapter 2.)

Religious belief is less evident. Patients and doctors may unwittingly alienate one another with a chance remark. Offering a termination of pregnancy to a devout Catholic may be deeply offensive. Indeed, some doctors themselves refuse to deal with termination requests on religious grounds, handing over such cases to their agnostic partners.

It is unreasonable to expect doctors and patients to know the intricate details of every religion. But it is reasonable for them to explore their belief systems. It may be that the Asian patient facing the doctor is a liberal Muslim. She may want to be treated as a 'Western' patient. She may, however, become deeply disturbed should she find herself in the company of a male doctor and particularly if he closes the door or tries to perform a simple examination. It is the responsibility of such a patient to try and make her or his views understood. If she is too frightened to explain them, it is the doctor's responsibility to define the patient's beliefs before proceeding. It is often difficult to do so in the hurly-burly of general practice, and especially if there are language problems (see Chapter 2). However, doctors do need to be aware of each patient's religious beliefs and so avoid inappropriate behaviour. Time must be set aside and interpreters called in if necessary.

When it comes to treatment, particular care must be taken. One patient I assumed to be a Hindu announced he was a Jain, a Buddhist-like religion for whom the central code of conduct is non-violence to any living creature. I was not clear whether this would extend to infestations like lice and fleas, but fortunately I never needed to find out. In some religious festivals, particularly among Orthodox Jews and Muslims, taking anything by mouth is forbidden between sunrise and sunset. Essential medicines may have to be taken at night or special dispensation obtained from the religious adviser in the event of an emergency. Similarly, the treatment itself carries risk of religious offence. Capsules containing gelatin and some pills containing milk products might offend an Orthodox Jew. The Muslim patient's resistance to take the pills might well be that the medicines were passed to the patient in the doctor's left hand. For Muslims, the left hand is reserved for washing, particularly the genital and anal areas, and the right hand reserved for food and anything passed to the mouth.

Hindus consider a woman's monthly period to be a time when she is unclean. She should avoid the preparation of food at this time. Imagine the disturbance to family life, then, if a Hindu mother was unable to prepare food for her daughter's wedding because of the doctor's insistence on starting a hormone therapy at a particular time.

Death, too, carries a stigma in many religions. For Hindus it is particularly disturbing to have been in contact with a dead body without the ritual washing and prayers. Many would not be happy to be examined by a doctor who had recently attended a death.

The key to all these situations is for patient and doctor to sit down together and establish where exactly the beliefs start and finish.

For a Jehovah's Witness the issue is particularly important. In the event of a risk to life from blood loss, the Witness would expect to be allowed to die. Many doctors would not be prepared to watch this happen and would try, especially in the case of a child, to get a Court Order to enforce treatment. This issue should be explored early in the patient–doctor relationship so there is no doubt where each party stands.

As doctors we are often exposed to unacceptable attitudes: the anti-Semitic remark made by a white Anglo-Saxon; the pejorative remarks about homosexuality or sexist attitudes to women and men. Some of these attitudes will be found in doctors as I'm sure we can be just as prejudiced as any other group. Presumably there are racist doctors and patients who find each other and are happy.

Similarly, there may be born-again Christians, nuclear disarmers, communists and fascists happily agreeing with each other in the surgery. But this is often not the case, and even with the best training available doctors' and patients' beliefs will get in the way of the consultation. Some of the most rewarding experiences in looking after patients has been where each other's beliefs have been acknowledged and respected. This acknowledgement and respect seems to be a factor at the heart of family medicine and one which must be preserved (see Chapter 3).

Looking back over the last 15 years, I can think of some examples to support this: the bedsit birth of a baby boy to cockney White Muslims. Their quiet prayers as the barefoot midwife wrapped the baby; the look of total peace on the Tamil priest's face as I tried to convince him that he should worry about his physical health; the devotion of a young man to his partner dying from AIDS. The sick man was too weak to stand, so his partner would carry him to the bath or toilet, unwilling to let anyone else help him.

Honesty

Why do we all lie? Is it to save embarrassment for ourselves or others? Is it because we would cause more pain with truth? Or is it just a lazy habit that's easy?

Doctors' lies

Taking blood
Just a little scratch now.

> Truth: I'm going to put a needle in your arm, it sometimes hurts.

Giving pills
Take them after food, they sometimes upset the stomach.

> Truth: These can cause a haemorrhage from the stomach, especially if you haven't eaten. There is a small chance it could be fatal.

Examining patients
You've just got a couple of bruised ribs, they're not cracked.

> Truth: I don't know whether they're broken or not. It doesn't make any difference as the treatment is the same. But I want to sound as if I really can tell the difference.

For doctors, lying or using a 'medical euphemism' is usually to cover insecurity or to support professional status that seems under attack. The truth may mean admitting grievance and accepting errors. These are difficult areas for doctors whose training tends to discourage self-disclosure and professional openness. As training goes on, the doctor will have faced nightmare stories and horrific sights. One way to survive will be to stay in 'control' and not show any distress. The pain gets kept inside and the outer skin is thickened. Eventually the doctor is fooled into thinking he or she can cope with anything. This confidence breeds respect from frightened patients. The cycle grows until a mistake is made. The mistake may subconsciously 'tune in' to a vulnerable doctor's core and the doctor will find it difficult to climb down, fearing a breakdown. The communication that follows may be artificial. The patient may sense the doctor is not telling the whole truth and become suspicious not only of the one remark but also of behaviour generally.

For the doctor to tell the truth, even if admitting ignorance, can be particularly comforting for patients. They sometimes feel the person in front of them is human after all and has problems like anyone else. If interest in the patient's situation continues and a willingness to find out what is not known is expressed, then the relationship is often improved. The doctor's openness is likely to encourage patients to do the same.

Patients' lies

Alcohol

Oh, very little. I drink about a glass of wine a day with my evening meal.

Truth: I must do someting about reducing my drinking, beer with lunch, half a bottle of wine in the evenings. That's more than 40 units a week.

Backs

I must have done my back lifting a cabinet at work. I'll need a certificate.

Truth: My mum's ill and everyone else takes time off sick at the office, why not me? That boss is such a mean bastard.

Relationships

We've been happily married for 13 years.

Truth: He's been cheating on me for 3 years but I haven't got the energy to fight for him any more.

Not telling the truth can obviously cause problems, particularly where medicines and treatments are being given. If there has been no improvement with a treatment, the doctor might double the dosage of the medicine hoping for a cure. If the original dose was not taken as prescribed, such an action is dangerous. Similarly, lies get recorded in medical records and might be acted on at a later date.

My husband always takes a few of my sleeping pills.

Truth: I need *more* just at the moment.

or worse

There's no way I could have caught VD. I've been faithful.

Truth: There's no way I could tell *her*.

or worse still

No, I've never had an epileptic fit.

Truth: I've just *got* to get this HGV (Heavy Goods Vehicle) licence.

Patient and Doctor Expectations

Some patients and their doctors see their relationship in terms of uncomplicated body mechanics: some part of the body or mind is malfunctioning and needs amending or repairing. This view can be satisfying for both as the doctor feels like the skilled mechanic with a job to do and the patient gets a problem sorted out without unnecessary fuss. Many patient–doctor interactions work like this and both may be totally satisfied.

Problems can arise if the 'mechanic' starts to point out that the damage is caused by the way the body has been 'driven' or that the damage is too severe to be repaired. The patient may expect that damage can always be repaired even if the 'body' is old and has never been properly cared for. The patient may feel that his 'mechanic' is just not giving the right advice and may seek another opinion.

If doctors can only work in the mechanic mode they will tend to attract patients who share this approach. And they will alienate patients who seek a deeper understanding of their lives and their situation.

Similarly, if doctors can only work in philosopher mode, seeking deeper meanings in every interaction, they will alienate patients who seek simple pragmatic answers.

What would seem to be needed is an ability to change modes not only to each end of the scale described above, but also to the infinite variations in between. Finding out what expectations are present in each patient–doctor interaction is difficult and can be time-consuming. But if it is not explored it can cause serious problems.

Here is a simple consultation about a rash:

P: Hello Doctor, I'm back again with this rash.
Thinks: Oh good, it is her again; at least she'll see the cream didn't work.

D: Oh hello, I wasn't expecting to see that rash again.
Thinks: Why hasn't it gone? I am sure it was fungal. Maybe he didn't use the cream or maybe he's really worried about something else.
Let's have a look.

P: You see, it hasn't changed much but it's spread to my legs now.
Thinks: She's looking puzzled. I bet she doesn't know what it is.

D: Yes, I can see what you mean; how often did you use the cream?
Thinks: He can't have used it properly.

P:　Twice a day, as you said, for ten days.
　　Thinks: She's looking more puzzled – oh god, maybe it's something dangerous.

D:　Well, we'll have to send some scrapings from the rash to the hospital to find out more about it.
　　Thinks: I'll prove it's a fungus then confront him about not using the cream.

P:　How long will that take?
　　Thinks: Oh no! I know it's dangerous, probably skin cancer at least – she looks really upset now, she probably knows how it will turn out.

D:　The tests will take a week or two, then we'll meet up to decide the best course of treatment for you.
　　Thinks: When he sees it in black and white he'll really use that cream properly.

P:　OK doctor.
　　Thinks: It's only a matter of time.

D:　Bye-bye.
　　Thinks: Why don't they do as we tell them?

This consultation may have taken only a few minutes. These few minutes have gone wrong and may leave the patient fearful for his life. It is likely that the patient and doctor left this consultation uncomfortable. Both will have picked up unease from the other, but they are not uneasy about the same things. The patient wanted a rash to be treated. The doctor wanted to be proved right. Neither got what they wanted or expected. This uncomfortable consultation, where neither's needs are met, is called 'dysfunctional' in general practice jargon. Dysfunctional consultations are common. In essence, patient and doctor have been failing to communicate clearly. There has been insufficient exploration and no negotiation, and there is unlikely to be shared reflection or objectives. Such dysfunctional consultations can be prevented by more exploration, more open questions, more examination of each other's beliefs.

In the short consultation about the rash the patient might

have said, 'Why do you think the rash hasn't gone?' or even, 'Do you think it's something serious?' The doctor may have asked the same questions. In either case the consultation would have changed and the fear of cancer and the suspicion of non-compliance would have been revealed.

The challenge for patients would seem to be the ability to be heard. The ability to show feelings and thoughts even with fear, embarrassment and anger. This will mean taking risks and the doctor must help to make it safe enough for those risks to be taken.

The challenge for general practitioners is to pick up the clues from the patients, to become an expert at listening, watching and thinking, to tailor make each response, prescription and action and in all this to be respectful of the patient's autonomy. I have made the assumption that the good general practitioner will already be a good diagnostician and expert on preventive health care. This is a tall order and in reality it is often different. The doctors may have had insufficient or disorganized training in these areas; they may have emotional or physical problems themselves, or just not have had enough sleep.

In these situations, the patients have to make the best of what they've got. Sometimes they can seek out other doctors or be prepared to confront the doctor with their needs and his/her shortcomings. It may come to a forced change of doctor or a formal complaint.

2 Difficulties

Embarrassment

We all get embarrassed and we can all think of something we
would rather not talk about with partners, friends or our
doctors. Some of these issues linger in our minds and affect our
concentration and daily functioning. Deciding to talk about it
may come only after nights of mounting fear and panic. Surgery
appointments may have been booked, cancelled and rebooked
before the chosen day. It may be the first time you have talked
about an incident to anyone. It is not uncommon for patients to
be unable to carry it through when faced with the real consultation. Some patients will 'test the water' with a minor complaint before disclosing what they have really come to discuss.
It is easy to forget that these minor complaints are often 'testers'
and it is difficult to maintain interest and sensitivity in the face
of what feels like trivia. The patient may have their hand on the
door before turning and saying: 'There was just one other thing
doctor . . .'

The issue in question may be anything: it may concern a
sexual incident of which we are ashamed, and we may need to
describe exactly what happened and with whom; we may want
to show the doctor a rash or a mole; we may have to face
thoughts or feelings which we had hoped to keep to ourselves.

We may be embarrassed by some aspect of our personality or
some part of our body, or perhaps being caught unwell and

unwashed. There are many embarrassing situations that are commonly faced by patients. And, as if this is not enough, patients may be faced with a doctor or other professional of whom the sex, personality, culture or attitude makes it more difficult to speak openly. Some patients will prefer to visit a doctor they know well, others will seek out a stranger. Family doctors may be too close for comfort. The patient sensing that, despite trusting the doctor's confidentiality, the link to relatives and friends somehow remains. Facing an embarrassing situation now may mean a reminder of that moment at every future contact.

In the sections that follow, the focus is on sex, physical examination, self-image, hygiene and sexual orientation. These are only examples; the causes of embarrassment are too numerous to describe.

Embarrassment about Sex

Film censors judge which film is suitable for which age group. However, a '15' or '18' rating gives no idea to the public just which bits were felt suitable or unsuitable. Some might feel that a violence, sex or embarrassment rating in addition would help parents and others decide on film choice. Such a rating for embarrassment or 'squirm' value could be applied to contact with doctors.

Patients' 'squirm' factor can be higher just thinking about the intimate sexual issues they will need to talk about in the surgery. These issues may have to be discussed with doctors who 'squirm' themselves when faced with explicit discussions about sex.

For example:

Doctor, I'm embarrassed to talk about this but . . .

My boyfriend wants anal intercourse with me. Does that mean he's a homosexual? Can I catch AIDS from this?

My girlfriend had herpes a few years ago. We always use a condom, but can I catch it if we have oral sex even if she hasn't got an attack?

or

> I've got a problem with my erection. The other night it just
> disappeared at the wrong moment. What can I do?

Questions like these often appear in the problem pages of
magazines. For many, an anonymous letter to an agony aunt or
uncle is easier than facing the doctor. This is partly because face-
to-face discussion would mean facing up to the problem generally, but it would also mean exposing oneself to the possibility
of rejection and prejudice from the doctor.

Some patients feel strong enough to confront the doctor who
seems not to listen or understand:

> Doctor, you seem shocked to hear I'm having an affair. Would
> you rather I talked about it to someone else?

> Look Doctor, I don't know how many gay men you look after but
> we are very careful these days – in fact more careful than most
> of my straight friends.

But more often the patient stays silent, sensing the unspoken
reproach.

> A young couple came to the surgery one evening. I had only
> seen them once before, shortly after their marriage six months
> earlier. I was struck by the change from the elated newly-weds I
> remembered to this tired and weathered pair. They both started
> talking at once and gradually it came out that they had been
> trying to start a family since their marriage. They wanted to know
> if they should worry after six months of trying. Were they
> normal? Would they have to adopt? I remarked that they
> certainly looked worried and then asked them if they would
> answer some personal questions about their sexual life together.
>
> My questions and their answers did not reveal a couple who
> had failed to consummate their marriage. Nor had they sexual
> difficulties of premature ejaculation, vaginismus, loss of erection,
> or pain on intercourse. Nor had they been putting the wrong bits
> together nor avoiding the right time.
>
> Instead they revealed a tired, misinformed start of a marriage.
> The wife explained that her nan had told her to concentrate love-

making at the beginning and end of her 'monthlies'. Her husband explained he had been conceived, as had all his brothers, when his mum had her periods. In addition to this family health mythology, they themselves used common sense and decided they should try as often as possible as this made it more likely. For six months they had dutifully made love daily and more at weekends until exhausted and dejected they came to the doctor.

Although daily intercourse is at one end of the normal range, this couple had concentrated their efforts at the least fertile times of the cycle. Somehow they had kept going with a growing sense of failure and managed to be still talking and loving one another despite the pressure. Such misinformation is common in families and only by exploring the beliefs will they be revealed. After discussing it they left feeling rather proud of themselves and some months later returned with some good news.

Jim lived in sheltered housing; he had given up his house when he had reached 70 as he couldn't manage the garden. He had always been single since losing a fiancée in the war and I know from photographs in his room he still thought of her. He certainly hadn't expected another relationship to come at his time of life.

He attended the surgery for arthritis in his knees and seemed to hover near the door unable to leave. He remarked, 'I suppose it's perverted for a man of my age to have sexual feelings.' He resisted the urge to talk further at that stage despite my entreaties to sit down, but did promise to talk at a future consultation.

Later he described years of mourning his girlfriend and hard dedication to his work. He had been surprised to be visited at home by a former colleague from work. She was in her late 50s and he had never realized she was fond of him. This relationship had grown and seemed to him threatened by his bungled attempt at intercourse. His sense of guilt and failure had prevented him trying again.

During the consultation he would frequently exclaim that he shouldn't be here talking to the doctor about such things, and how ashamed he felt discussing it at all.

He would blush when asked to describe exactly what they did together and how it felt. He was shocked to hear about the frequency of intercourse in young couples and the normality of masturbation. With time his confidence grew and he explained that although he had a good erection at the start of lovemaking, it would disappear as he came near to penetration. He was convinced he was 'past it' and there was no hope for this improper relationship. He admitted that he woke from sleep with erections and was surprised to hear that the loss of erection prior to intercourse is usually a psychological problem, not a physical one.

He was further convinced when I encouraged him to prove it by masturbation. It had been the first time for many years and he returned youthful and triumphant.

Gradually he and his partner discussed their problem more openly and eventually they came to the surgery together to talk further. Their crushing embarrassment reminded me of the rare interviews with teenage lovers. Discussing the problem together they found that the responsibility was shared and the sexual problems gradually resolved. They appreciated why the problem had occurred and she talked of how much she had always wanted him. He expressed his sense of guilt and shame in 'soiling' the memory of his wartime fiancée and was able to show how much he wanted the new relationship.

In the surgery doctors can only explore sexual issues to the limit of their own defences and to the limit of their own taboos. Consultations where a confident patient talks about explicit sexual issues to an inhibited doctor are fraught with problems. Similarly, an open, uninhibited doctor can unwittingly inhibit a shy patient. Respect for each other is best established first and, as discussed in Chapter 1, the 'personal contract' may not extend to such a subject.

Embarrassment about Physical Examination

Taboos about clothing and nakedness are part of every culture. As a doctor I am exposed to a range of behaviour in the course of physical examinations. At one end of the range a Muslim woman veiled in a yashmak, chaperoned and asking for a female doctor and at the other end a barely dressed Westerner on a summer's day.

What is acceptable in any culture is dependent on the situations and circumstances. The English might feel comfortable in swimwear at the beach or swimming pool, but would probably cringe at the idea of semi-nakedness in church. Such social codes of behaviour also exist in doctors' surgeries.

An American woman came in for a 'pap smear'. She had been asked at reception whether she would prefer a woman doctor or the nurse to do this examination. She said she was not particularly bothered either way. The test, our equivalent of a cervical smear, would usually be done in a gynaecologist's office as the concept of family doctor is uncommon in the USA.

I noted the surprise on the woman's face as she came through the door. She explained that she had expected a doctor in a white coat and tie. When it came to the examination, she was shocked to find there were no stirrups on the examination couch. American doctors routinely use them but they appear barbaric to many English doctors and patients. My homely surgery had been designed to put anxious or troubled patients at ease. Instead, for her, it lacked the clinical, efficient and scientific atmosphere of her gynaecologist's office. Despite this, she decided to go through with the test and then talked about the different expectations of each country and each patient.

Sometimes the embarrassment isn't the patient's, it's the doctor's:

I remember being troubled by a young woman who arrived in early pregnancy. She sat down in my consultation room as I asked her for some details of the pregnancy. As I wrote these down I mentioned she would need to be weighed. She got up and before I had realized had undressed and jumped on the weighing scales. As she stood there I was flummoxed. What should I do or say? The options whirred through my mind. Do I ask her why she felt it was all right to pad around the consultation room undressed? Supposing I was to suggest she might be cold and to put something on? Or should I just carry on as if it happened every day?

In the end I chose the latter – probably preferring not to appear a prude rather than because of sound professional judgement. At the time there was no hint of self-consciousness in the patient nor sign of intended sexual messages. Was I fooling myself that this situation was without embarrassment for her. *I* was certainly embarrassed and felt uneasy about my ability to handle it. My mind whirred again, why was I embarrassed? After all, in the course of a first antenatal visit I would be expected to examine heart and breasts, tummy and vagina. But this patient had not chosen to stand behind the curtain and undress piecemeal. As I thought of these things my colleague Linda, the community midwife, walked in. The patient made no effort to cover herself and held out a hand in introduction. As the pregnancy progressed she continued to be uninhibited by our standards, whether with male or female doctors. Furthermore, there was no change when her husband joined her in the clinic nor when she was in labour itself.

In situations such as this it is the doctor who is embarrassed. We are taught to protect ourselves by inviting chaperones for examinations. We are also taught to give simple specific messages when it comes to physical examination. A doctor who can say 'You need to take off your trousers and underpants' gives the confident message that he has been in the situation before. A half-hearted 'You need to take some things off' may finish up with an embarrassed patient and doctor. Similarly, a doctor facing an embarrassed person of the opposite sex needs to ask 'What do you find embarrassing?' and 'What would make it less embarrassing?'

Looking back I realize I missed the opportunity to discuss the uninhibited woman's beliefs and values. How had she come to behave in the way she did? Was it a family trait? Did she grow up in a country where nakedness was the norm? I should have asked her to explain how it was she was unaware of the more usual social codes. Perhaps I would have discovered an anger about convention and a dedicated belief to confront it; I may also have discovered evidence of sexual enjoyment in watching professionals look uncomfortable, but then again I may not have.

This experience was a valuable lesson, it taught me to identify where my boundaries (see p. 76) were in the area of embarrassment and physical examination. Each doctor has his or her own social code for what is acceptable in this area. When the patient steps outside this code it is time to stop and confront the situation. To do so will be to avoid the possibility of litigation; it also leaves the patient in no doubt about what is acceptable and what is not; and it allows the patient to confront what is acceptable for her or him.

Examining the genitals

Part of the physical examination means examining the genitals. For doctors of sex opposite to the patient's it poses a difficult problem. How can they examine a vagina or penis in a neutral way? Will the patient receive this examination without a hint of sexual overtones? For a heterosexual male doctor it is easy to examine the penis in a neutral way. Similarly, heterosexual female doctors can examine a vagina without giving it undue respect or contempt. However, when these doctors approach the examination of a patient of the opposite sex they bring with them not only their medical training and experience, which may be limited, but also their own sexual experience which may be even more limited.

Does the woman doctor fumbling over an examination of a penis reveal herself as just an inexperienced doctor or as an inexperienced lover as well?

When discussing these situations with other doctors it can cause embarrassment and a surprising range of behaviour for professionals who have to conduct examinations daily. My close friends, a husband and wife in general practice partnership together, were discussing this subject with me after dinner. I asked my male colleague whether he would warm instruments such as a speculum before inserting them into the vagina. He replied that of course he would as it was a normal courtesy. His wife was shocked, she felt that as a woman she would receive a warm speculum as one full of sexual messages and insisted a cold speculum indicated to the patient that this was a clinical examination. He protested that a cold speculum was cruelty, but then had to retreat when she asked him would he warm an instrument for examining the rectum (a proctoscope). The fact that this heterosexual doctor had been warming specula for 10 years in practice yet never thinking of warming a proctoscope exposes his sexuality in routine physical examinations. I am left uncertain. Cruel or sexually provocative, perhaps room temperature for both is best.

Clearly, the doctor brings his or her history of sexuality to the consultation. It helps to be aware of this as it is the doctor's primary duty to be aware of the patient's history and behaviour. The doctor who has not yet worked out his or her own codes of conduct in this area is not in a position to help patients effectively. Increasingly, doctors practise in partnerships, and, fortunately, many of those partners are women. It becomes increasingly likely that as patients talk to doctors, and doctors talk to each other, their range of acceptable behaviour is established.

Where the patient has sexual difficulties, they may be referred to a doctor who is psychosexually trained. This training usually lasts four years and is hoped to allow the doctor to explore the patient's difficulties without any influence from the doctor's sexuality:

One patient consulted repeatedly with an itchy penis. He would come in to the consultation room and with barely a word start to show me his penis. He would stand in front of me, suck in his tummy and lift his penis out of the top of his trousers. He treated his penis with contempt, dragging it upwards by its foreskin and cruelly prodding the area concerned. I felt it was easy to comment that he was treating his penis as an enemy. I wondered if a woman doctor would be able to say this in the same situation. In any event it transpired that he was angry with his penis for letting him down. He and his partner had an unhappy sexual life for which he blamed himself. As a consequence, his penis was rarely washed and I'm sure felt neglected.

The man and his partner were referred to a psychosexual doctor together and his consultations with me for a sore penis promptly stopped.

It was my first day as a student on the wards; we had been taught to take blood from patients. As we got our lists of patients we disappeared to 'bleed' them one by one. My first few patients predictably mentioned Dracula and were friendly and encouraging. I then proceeded to a curtained bed occupied by a blowsy middle-aged woman. As I was taking her blood she 'accidently' revealed herself from under the sheets. She asked if I would like to slip in for a quick cuddle. I was shocked and deeply embarrassed. At a time when it was so important to look professional and competent here was a patient destroying my composure. Part of this embarrassment was a failure to be taught about ways to deal with these situations. The teachers I had did not acknowledge there was a problem: they appeared not to be in tune with the patient's or their own sexual feelings.

At no time as a medical student was I taught how to deal effectively with situations full of embarrassment. We were just taught the mechanics of medicines as if these issues didn't arise. It didn't take long to discover where the truth lay. Later on, when training for general practice, we would discuss how these situations can be handled. One experienced family doctor admitted he used to bring the conversation 'back to reality' by asking if the patient had an offensive vaginal discharge or how often he or she had diarrhoea. This crude method was his answer to stemming any hint of sexuality. He used this method as he wanted to avoid a direct confrontation with the patient. Such a confrontation, however, can leave the patient in no doubt of the doctor's position and his or her ability to face it. Of course, to get such confidence one must have already confronted one's own sexual feelings and have examined carefully any tendency to encourage sexual approaches from patients.

Embarrassment about Self Image

Patients sometimes joke about being caught with dirty underwear or socks with holes in them. These jokes have a ring of
truth for all of us. I went on a course some years ago to study
osteopathy. The lecturer announced to the group of doctors that
now his introduction was over we would all be involved in
practical demonstrations. He asked us to strip down to our
underwear. Looking around the room there were plenty of
pants with holes in, frayed bras and old knickers. The following
day the same group arrived and this time there was a sea of
smart and fashionable underwear.

In the surgery the patients' self image is often under threat.
The doctor may have to see the obese abdomen, the hairy back
or the spotty bottom. Most of us are embarrassed about some or
other facet of our self image. One particular patient had never
taken her underwear off in changing rooms. She avoided the
seaside and covered up in summer, saying she got a rash in the
sun. In fact, she had never undressed as an adult in another
person's company, unless the lights were dimmed. Her concern
was dark hair on the inside of her thighs and around her
nipples. A woman doctor examined her and sensitively shared
how common body hair is in women. She also helped her look
at her prejudice about other people's body image. This woman,
with such strong feelings about her appearance, admitted she
could not stand the idea of men with beards or moustaches.

It is quite common for patients to make a remark in the
course of a routine examination: 'As you can see I'm not very
well endowed' or 'I'm very flat chested' or 'I'm embarrassed
about my stretch marks.' This is a difficult area and it is easy for
the doctor to find himself thinking or saying, 'You look very
normal or perfectly all right to me.' But it is perhaps more
helpful to get the patient to describe how she or he has come to
see herself as she does. Who was it that made the remark that
hurt her and who is she comparing herself to?

Others are embarrassed by the change in their bodies. Perhaps
the surgical scar on their abdomen that with age has left an
impression of tethered cloth. Alternatively, the burn across one

shoulder which remains hidden, or the bald pate covered by a wig or hat.

More commonly it is embarrassment about the effects of age on our bodies. The spidery veins that gradually appear on the thighs, the 'crow's feet' around the eyes or the fat that mysteriously just seems to arrive.

For the patient coming to the doctor it must be difficult to remember that doctors see the complete range of human size and shape. The patient's concern about his image rarely matches the reality of his situation. However, looking at his concern seriously does remind him that he is still worthwhile as a person. Looking at the distress and embarrassment can help the patients deal with their feelings in a way that plastic surgery often can't.

Embarrassment about Hygiene

How would it feel to find out that others avoid you? They may have noticed your bad breath or body odour. Perhaps you smell of urine as your control is not as it was. Most of us would like someone to tell us – hopefully someone cares enough to face us with it.

In the surgery I suspect most of us are more concerned to clear the air with air freshener or open windows so that the next patient doesn't think the smell is coming from us. It's embarrassing to face another person and tell him he smells, and easier to avoid it. An honest observation may be taken with offence but more likely with gratitude.

One patient kept her shoes on throughout her pregnancy. She made the excuse that it would take too long to undo the double knots. I noticed as time passed she chose boots and shoes with elaborate laces or thongs up the leg. Eventually in labour she confessed to having smelly feet. It dominated her life and affected her relationships. She washed regularly but found even new shoes soon became 'contaminated'. Help was available for her, as there are some effective treatments, but she had not felt confident enough to get it.

Often the embarrassment is the doctor's: the patient may live in damp surroundings and have no money for cleaning clothes. To pass comment would appear insensitive, especially when the doctor is likely to be so much better provided for.

Often hygiene issues arise where there is no fault in the patient: the mentally ill man coming in for his injection unaware of soiled underwear; the elderly man who dribbles urine and stains his trousers. These patients cannot help themselves and need resources and respect. Somehow doctors need to overcome inhibitions and try to care for them as if the hygiene issue wasn't there.

I am embarrassed to think of the number of times I have avoided examining patients who smelled or were filthy. It's easy to rationalize that an examination would be unlikely to contribute to the diagnosis and treatment.

Embarrassment about Sexual Orientation

When new patients come to the surgery it is part of the doctor's brief to ask about past and family illnesses, home situation and relationships. For this to be done successfully, the doctor must have come to terms with his or her own attitudes to sexual orientation. No matter how the questions are asked, the patient will sense the doctor's position.

Doctor A: Hello Mrs Smith, thank you for filling in our questionnaire. I see you have no serious family or past medical illnesses. You're staying near the station, is that a flat? Do you have a boyfriend or fiancé? Does he live with you?

Doctor B: Hello Carol, it's your first visit here isn't it? Sorry about the questionnaire, but it helps us to get to know our patients. I see mum and dad are fit and well and you've been lucky with your health. Are you on your own in the flat? Do you use contraception?

Doctor C: Hello, I'm Doctor . . . You've just registered haven't you? How do you like to be addressed, Mrs, Miss, Ms? Before you tell me why you've come today, can I ask you some

personal details? I see from the questionnaire you and your
family have had good health. What about relationships? Do you
have a sexual relationship at the moment? Are you heterosexual
or homosexual? Does your partner live with you?

The patient may feel comfortable with any of these three
doctors. Most, I think, would prefer Doctor C to Doctors A or B
as more responsibility stays with the patient and she (in this
case) might feel that respect would be shown no matter what
her sexual orientation might be. If the start goes well then
patients may go on to discuss sensitive issues without
embarrassment.

Despite more than 10 years of facing these situations, I still
feel clumsy grappling for words to ask questions in 'squirm'
situations. I was certainly helped by a number of remarkable
patients who showed no embarrassment in discussing the most
difficult subjects. How easy it is to proceed when the person
you're talking to shows clearly that there are no taboo areas.

One patient who helped me was Chrissy, an actress, who at the
first interview announced she was a transsexual. She was
awaiting her gender operation to remove her penis and testicles.
She wanted further supplies of female hormone that would
remove body hair and maintain breast development. Even her
agent did not know she was a transsexual and she explained
she taped her genitals underneath her for the more explicit
outfits. She waited patiently and finally went through with her
operation. A traumatic post-operative time followed where,
despite being quite ill, she managed to maintain her new vagina
with the glass dilators she was given. Eventually she married a
man who knew about her secret and they moved abroad.

Chrissy's ability to talk about anything without embarrassment
was in sharp contrast to the measured society conversations
that are more normal in the surgery. Her openness at times felt
vulgar and uninhibited, but I knew it was mainly my prejudice.
Gradually it has become easier to talk to patients about their
sexuality, their relationships and their inhibitions which make
up so much of human suffering.

Embarrassment about Showing Emotion

The woman was crying. Through the tears she said how much she hoped she wouldn't cry this time. She had waited outside in the waiting room feeling quite relaxed but once through the door it had all 'gone wrong'. It was in contrast with her image of herself and she hated the idea that she might be thought of as the sort of woman who could cry in the doctor's surgery. On listening to her it was clear that there was nowhere else to cry. Her husband had been told he had a heart condition and she was careful to avoid upsetting him. Her father had died a year ago and her mother was still grieving. She taught at a secondary school and the staff room seemed hostile. I thought her husband might have sensed her emotions anyway even though she thought she was hiding them well. She disagreed and decided to stay away from the surgery as it embarrassed her to cry and because she thought she just needed to keep going.

I visited a charming elderly man whose wife had just died. We talked about how he was managing without her and he broke down and sobbed. Later, as I was leaving, he said, 'I am sorry I made such a fool of myself, it's just that I miss her so much.'

'Letting go' or 'breaking down' is still seen as a sign of weakness and a cause for embarrassment. Often we say 'Go on have a good cry, it'll do you good', but we may be thinking 'Don't make *too* much noise' or '*You* may cry in this situation but I wouldn't.'

I sometimes say to patients who are embarrassed that they should consider their emotions a gift. Just as they are likely to feel the depth of despair or fire of anger, they also are more likely to feel heights of joy and passion. I'm not sure I've convinced anybody, least of all myself, and when you're in the middle of it you feel that any other way must be better.

It's not always the patient that gets embarrassed. I remember a woman saying, 'I feel like shouting and screaming when I think of what he's done to me.' I replied, 'Why don't you?' I expected a measured reply but she just sat there and screamed and screamed without stop. I was dumbstruck and after a while my partners came in to see what was happening. I felt the situation was out of control and was embarrassed to be checked up on, but in fact the woman was *gaining* control of her situation; did what she *had* to do: express how she felt. I gave her permission to do so, and so shouldn't have been surprised at all.

Some situations are embarrassing as one gets caught out wearing the wrong emotion. My father, a doctor too, used to tell a true story about a particularly tiresome and talkative patient:

> The patient seemed never to listen to his advice and would constantly interrupt with her own ideas. She continued to visit him over the years and I sensed she was more than a match for him. One day, after moving into new consulting rooms, he endured another half an hour with her. As she got up to leave she headed for the wrong door. He got up to protest but she stopped him as usual. Impulsively, she opened the door and descended head over heels into the basement. The ambulance arrived and took her to hospital with many broken bones. Later he noticed her footprint on the ceiling of the steep staircase to the basement. Over the next 20 years he would retell the story at every opportunity and convulse with laughter at this tragedy. On many occasions friends and acquaintances would be shocked that a doctor could have such feelings and strange emotions.

Having inherited a similar sense of humour I have been on the lookout for such situations:

> On one occasion, when attending a birth in hospital, my partner was caught out. The baby had been safely delivered by the midwife and the woman was being stitched up by my partner. Just then the husband stood up and felt very faint. The midwife, an experienced 56-year-old grandmother, rushed over to catch him. Unfortunately, he fell, cracking his head and landing on her. He was unconscious. She was trapped, panicked and she developed chest pains. The husband was admitted to hospital

with his head injury and the midwife admitted with angina, both were still in hospital when mother and baby went home.

Doctors together often laugh about real tragedies; their 'sick' sense of humour is common. It is a defence, of course, against the pain of listening to tales of suffering day in and day out. It's only one of the ways the doctor's engine keeps running, thus helping to prevent early 'burn out'.

Checklist for the Fearful/Embarrassed Patient

1   Remember that however difficult the problem, it is likely that the doctor has encountered something similar with other patients.
2   Choose the doctor you feel most comfortable with.
3   Start with: 'I've got something that I'm very *afraid/ embarrassed* to talk about . . .'
4   Be prepared to tell the whole story and to tell the complete truth as this will help greatly.
5   If the doctor appears unhelpful it is not because you are unhelpable, just that the doctor has difficulties in dealing with your problem (see p. 100). Ask where you can get further help with your problem.

Fear

It seems to be a natural attendant to things medical: feeling ill is frightening; doctors are frightening, their pills, potions, tests and operations are fearful; the medical world is mysterious, full of ritual and secret behaviours. Entering that world, patients face leaving the world they know, trusting doctors and risking never returning to normal. This fear is in every consultation; in particular it revolves around some common themes.

Fear of Death

Most of us seem to live life as if we will live forever. The outrage in many patients when faced with a serious illness reflects this attitude. Patients will often say 'But I have always been so

healthy!' or 'My stomach/heart/lungs have always been my
strong part!' It is almost with disgust in their voice that they
protest and want to reject the diagnosis. Once the shock and the
mourning for our health is past, there is often a period of
adjustment to the new image of oneself. At this time, many
patients like to sit down in the surgery to discuss life expectancy
and the nature of the likely final illness.

Life Expectancy (%) for men and women

Age	Male	Female
0	71.7	77.5
15	57.8	63.4
30	43.4	48.7
45	29.2	34.3
60	16.7	21.1
75	7.9	10.4

Few patients will have the outlook of one elderly lady whom I
used to care for.

This lady, on finding her chest X-ray showed cancer of the lung,
booked in to see me to discuss her impending death. Over
several weeks she read about the complications of treatment
and explored the likely symptoms and signs that might develop.
As she got more breathless and was confined to bed by her
disease, she asked for sufficient medicines to keep her free from
the distress of breathlessness. I remember one conversation
when she clarified what dose of her morphine would relieve
breathlessness and what dose would stop her breathing.
   Death itself held no fear for her, but she was determined to
have control over her symptoms until the last. When she died in
her sleep her bottle of medicine had been spilt beside the bed
and I was never sure whether it was she who had decided the
time had come.

This attitude is unusual. Most patients and doctors seem to
prefer to travel hopefully, as if being too definite about the facts
would hasten their arrival. It takes a special relationship
between patient and doctor for death to be an easy area for
conversation.

Doctors are taught to ask open-ended questions to define the patient's perception of his or her illness. These questions cannot be answered 'Yes' or 'No', but require an answer that exposes what the person thinks. For example: 'What do you understand is wrong with you?' 'How do you view the future?' 'Looking ahead, what are you looking forward to?' 'If ever you were told you wouldn't get better, where would you want to be?' 'What frightens you most about your illness?' 'What are your religious beliefs?'

Rarely, open questions get asked by the patient; 'What will happen to me?' 'Will I get better from this?' 'How will I die?' 'How do you see it ending?' 'If you were me, what would you do now?'

Many relatives believe that loved ones would be best cared for in a state of ignorance. They have perhaps grown up with a parent who always feared death. They ask the doctor not to tell the patient what's wrong. But it is my experience that the patient guesses quickly by the embarrassed looks and furtive glances and the truth usually comes out.

Telling the 'truth' about dying doesn't always go right.

> A patient once pressed me to guess how long he might have to live now that his terminal illness had been diagnosed. On the strength of my replies he made important changes in his life, and now years later his illness shows no sign of deteriorating. Fortunately, he makes jokes about this conversation and bears no grudge, but I imagine how it could have been.

A doctor may face a similar situation when, having encouraged the family to come home to their dying father now at death's door, the patient rallies and lasts a further six months. Perhaps it is better to get it wrong than never to take the chance and leave family and patient guessing and regretting. Better still is to say: 'I don't know' or 'Who can tell these things?'

Exploring this taboo area usually leaves the patient and the doctor relieved. Often the fear of dying is something that is easy to relieve. Perhaps the patient thinks that he or she will be in agony or will haemorrhage. Frequently, patients fear being alone or fear being so confused as to say things they don't mean.

The doctor may be frightened the patient is going to ask for a terminal injection or blame the profession for his illness.

Fear of AIDS

A young man came to see me with a sore throat. I explained that his sore throat was caused by a virus. 'What sort of virus?' he asked. I explained that there were so many I couldn't possibly tell which one. He then surprised me by saying 'I couldn't have AIDS could I doctor?' He hadn't had unprotected intercourse with a partner he didn't know well, nor had he shared needles. In fact, it turned out that he had come into contact with sweat. When going to the gym for weight training three times a week he had noticed the equipment was wet from sweat and although he wiped it off he had begun to think about AIDS. As he exercised he imagined the AIDS virus creeping through his skin. Now weeks later he felt tired and had been sleeping poorly.

I reassured the young man but wondered how he would ever summon the courage to face a sexual relationship.

I seem to see a mixture of patients: those who are frightened about AIDS in their work and social lives, and those who recklessly put themselves at risk from catching the virus.

One heterosexual man who admitted that he had many sexual partners believed he 'moved too fast for the AIDS virus to catch me'.

A young homosexual man described how AIDS had decimated his friends and now he wasn't prepared to take any risks. He remarked that his sexual life felt at an end as no one was interested in oral sex whilst wearing a condom even if it was flavoured.

Some patients remember their first sexual encounters with great romance. In ignorance they discovered each other without particular threat. Now it has all changed, there is no room for ignorance, young people must know the risks, and in detail. Young men and women must overcome their inhibitions and carry condoms. They must insist their partners wear them.

Parents, teachers and doctors must be prepared to talk about AIDS and sex without embarrassment so that the myths are dispelled and the facts known.

Fear of Cancer

Fear of cancer is extremely common. When we are ill it is often cancer that seems the most likely cause of everyday symptoms. All patients (and especially doctors and nurses) are apt to say, 'I've had the headache for more than a week. You can guess what I think it is [brain tumour].' 'I've lost blood from the bowel. I think bowel cancer's in my family.' 'I've lost weight gradually over the last month. I look like Auntie Mary before she died of cancer.'

Some patients bring this fear into every consultation and every symptom. Sometimes the reason is obvious with a cruel memory of a loved one's lingering painful death. In other patients it is as if all life's worries are channelled into this one fear and they are never free of it. Reassurance is usually inappropriate as no amount of testing can pick up every early cancer. The best seems to be a mutual acknowledgement that the fear is there and there is a limit to how much to do.

Doctors usually fall into the trap of trying to reassure the patient before the true facts are available. I remember saying that I was certain that a breast lump was not cancer only to find after the biopsy that this was not the case. My own need to reassure this patient overtook caution and made her future care more difficult. To avoid this we must leave many terrified patients needlessly worried by obvious non-worrying lumps. What actually happens is that doctors play the odds: 'In my experience lumps like these are benign but just very rarely they're not.'

We have recently been told that 90 per cent of people who die from cancer of the neck of the womb (cervix) have never had a smear. How can one understand patients avoiding such a simple test that detects early cancer? How can we understand what makes a patient ignore a lump in the breast even though it's started to gnaw its way through the skin or even started to smell? Such denial often annoys doctors and the patients' relatives. It feels like a failure: failure not to have seen the patient years ago before it got so bad; failure not to be more approachable; failure in our education. Doctors don't like failing; they are a competitive bunch and it doesn't feel good to fail.

Surprisingly, 'denial' may be good for you. One study showed that women who denied they ever had cancer (despite having been told the diagnosis) did quite as well in surviving it as those who took an optimistic accepting outlook. Only those who got depressed were more likely to die earlier than the other two groups. I wonder what happens if you persuade deniers to face up to the health risks and responsibilities. Perhaps they shift into the depressed group and are more vulnerable to illness.

As cancers become easier to treat and more patients live successfully with them, maybe the fear will fade. In reality much of the fear is 'justified' as it *is* the commonest cause of death and for many fear of cancer is fear of death.

Fear of Heart Disease

Barely a week goes past in the surgery without seeing an apparently fit young man with chest pain. Sometimes he will have 'tested the water' first with a complaint such as wax in the ears or verrucae on the feet. Then, ashen-faced, he may describe left-sided chest pain and say, 'Do you think it's my heart?' Occasionally a father or uncle has had angina or a heart attack. Sometimes he will be bent over clutching his chest and breathing shallowly. Most often these symptoms in young men are associated with the muscles or cartilage joints of the rib cage. Finding the tender spot helps them to realize it's not their heart that's the problem. Occasionally its cause is the lining of the lung and the explanation of the 'catching pain' of this part of the lung will explain its knife-like quality that most of us have felt from time to time.

Patients are afraid of their symptoms; doctors are afraid of getting it wrong. Doctors know that perhaps once in their career they will come across the rare Wolff–Parkinson–White syndrome which causes irregular heart-beats. This complaint is diagnosed by an electronic tracing of heart-beats. Even if only one in 10,000 patients has the complaint, can we justify recommending ECG for all with an irregular heart-beat? Similarly, family doctors are on the lookout for the shortness of breath and pain on breathing that comes with air leaking from the lung (pneumothorax) or from blood clots travelling to the lung (pulmonary embolus). The first can be diagnosed by chest X-ray, and the second by lung scanning.

A family doctor can easily see patients who have chest pain on breathing, every week of their professional lives, but see cases of pneumothorax only every two or three years, and pulmonary embolus once in every five years.

Another common symptom is irregular heart-beats with a large gap afterwards. It is easy to understand the patient's feeling that the heart will stop at any moment. It is also difficult to persuade the patient to exercise and make the irregularity disappear, or to recognize the connection with stress or too much coffee.

So when patients visit the doctor with chest pain or palpitations, they hope to be told that all is well. They may expect their doctor to explain the possible causes and give some explanation as to why more serious illnesses are not likely. The doctor has to be tuned in to the physical presentation of the case, the full details of the complaint and to the circumstances in the patient's personal and working environment that may be relevant. The doctor also has to tune in to his/her own fear and make a balance of probabilities. Some types of chest pain should justify no further investigations or tests. Others should require careful examination and detailed investigation. Doctors, like most professionals, sometimes get it wrong.

A young man in his teens came to see me with palpitations. He described the attacks as if the heart was mis-timing. He was nervous in the surgery and on further discussion I gained an impression of an extremely anxious young man. He agreed the episodes seemed to come with anxiety and seemed content to wait and see if they settled. Eight years later he returned after many further attacks. He had got himself to hospital just as an attack started and at last his palpitations were diagnosed. Now on regular medicines, he is able to take more exercise and has had no further attacks. He is still an anxious young man and feels the attacks were worse when he was worried.

Fear of Disfigurement

What would you like to change about yourself? Is your nose too long or too short? What about your height or your weight? What about your breasts, your bottom, your belly, your double chin?

As a family doctor I frequently see patients who feel disfigured and would like to change something about themselves. Sometimes these feelings are part of a depression or other psychological disturbance, the symptom being the focus for a multitude of problems and difficult feelings. An attractive young woman might have come in to discuss the possibility of plastic surgery to remove a dimple on her face. It may be difficult to see how she would not be pleased to have such a dimple. Gradually it may become clear that to her the dimple is the cause of failed relationships and loss of confidence. Plastic surgeons are trained to carefully examine their patients' expectations to prevent disappointment and future litigation. However, plastic surgery can sometimes revolutionize the patients' feelings. I can think of a shy man with a large nose who became quite extrovert following his nose 'job'. Another patient, a woman, got her breast reduction on the NHS. She had deep strap marks in her shoulders from her bra and frequently complained of an aching back. After her operation although she had considerable scarring, to her the disfigurement was gone – she was able to run for a bus and swim without embarrassment.

Other patients endure disfigurement without comment. An elderly man accepted his colostomy and within hours of the operation understood about the changing of bags and their general care. For him to have survived the cancer operation was enough; he sensed his 'second chance' to live.

Others only wish they could have their old selves back. Burns, scars and more serious illnesses and accidents leave fear of disfigurement. Part of the recovery from such events is facing and coming to terms with the loss of our bodies as they were. Never being able to walk without a limp or play tennis as before.

Fear of Madness

It's there in so many of the consultations between patient and family doctor:

In the young parent
'If he doesn't stop crying I don't know what I'll do.'

In the depressed divorcee
'I can hear myself whining on – people don't want to hear it, I hate what I've become, I have got to get better. I don't know how to do it.'

In the adolescent
'I find myself thinking of dying, of car crashes and bloody accidents, is it normal?'

In the elderly
'I'm losing everything. I can't remember friends' names or even the family. At this rate I soon won't know anything.'

Madness or mental illness is common; there are few families without sufferers. Contrary to common belief only a few are unaware of their confusion and distress. Even in the elderly demented it is difficult to be sure that the previous personality of the patient is no longer suffering. Most patients remember their breakdowns or relapses and are acutely aware of their disturbance. It takes time for relatives and friends to accept them back into their lives and it is difficult too for the patient to feel confident of his or her own recovery. Where there is a family history of mental illness patients may be less frightened by the idea of their own psychiatric disturbance. Finding out that one's own mother suffered with depression after birth, for example, can be so reassuring to a new mother who feels alone with her depression and a baby.

Patients may suddenly see their anxiety as part of a family

'club' and be relieved. In my experience it is also common for the patient to be more afraid: they may fear 'finishing up like Aunt Mabel, who never got better' or 'like Uncle Charlie who tried to kill himself and got locked away'. Losing control of one's thoughts and feelings may also bring fear of 'electric treatment' or 'tranquillizer injections'.

Sometimes these patients are seen as the weak members in a family – and society – that never admits to emotional difficulties or mental distress. This idea of weakness is difficult to shift. In our society fighting pneumonia is acceptable, even heroic, but fighting depression is not.

Doctors often set a poor example, grasping the model of the overworked, caring doctor who is going to carry on until they drop. Often authoritative and dismissive, they are unable to see their own potential for illness and can only see it in their patients. This distancing elevates themselves and degrades the patient.

In reality this is far from the truth: doctors suffer with more mental illness than the average patient. They are more likely to be depressed and are more likely to kill themselves. Fortunately, things are changing and most young family doctors have been vocationally trained for the rigours of family practice. During this training the doctors are encouraged to examine their feelings and to accept the idea of their own emotional frailty. Acceptance of themselves as 'wounded healers' is of particular help with patients, especially those who fear mental illness. These young doctors can see the patient within themselves and are in touch with how it feels to be distressed. The patient in turn can sense this and is unlikely to leave feeling alone and rejected or misunderstood.

A doctor recently took over a patient from a colleague who has retired. The patient explained that he had known the doctor had suffered with depression for many years. When the patient developed his own depression he turned to his doctor for support and understanding. Together they explored the patient's symptoms at a depth that would only be possible with a fellow sufferer. Fortunately, the doctor was well enough to be able to do this and at no time did the patient feel he was looking after his doctor. The patient remembers it as an important experience and knows it will never be the same.

If this identification is too strong on either side then it loses its healing potential.

I find it helpful to think that we are all vulnerable to mental illness at any time. I have observed in myself, my patients and my colleagues that there are times when we are likely to become more like ourselves — more like exaggerations of our own personalities. I do not suffer with depression and 'low feelings' are always cured by sleep. My level of anxiety is sufficient to make me diligent and perhaps overwork, but not enough to bring my work home every night, nor to prevent sleep. Under stress my mental health fatigue emerges with obsessive behaviour. Already enjoying organizing and sorting problems, I become an obsessive list maker and compulsive analyser as life's pressures increase. Such self-disclosure to patients can help to diminish the fear of mental illness. It also helps me in my working life to acknowledge that I too can get ill and my friends and colleagues will tell me if they spot the signs.

Fear of Childbirth

'I made an awful noise didn't I? I was like an animal'.
'I'm going to split wide open if I push again'.
'I can't do it. I just can't do it'.
'I think the baby's dead, I can't feel it moving'.
'The pain was worse than anything I ever imagined'.

Women sometimes talk like this with their midwives and doctors, but more usually they talk to other women about these fears and experiences. It should be part of antenatal care to explore worries and concerns in pregnancy and the profession often forgets about this at the expense of measuring blood pressure, recording weight gain and testing urine.

In over a thousand women cared for in pregnancy, I can only think of a handful whose blood pressure was sufficiently high to disturb their pregnancy. I can, however, think of many women who had thought their babies were too active or not active enough; there have been hundreds who felt they'd make a fool of themselves in labour, or thought the baby would die; many regretted decisions they'd made and would do it differently next time.

Fear seems a normal part of the unknown. Reducing fear by exploring it is part of the midwives' and doctors' role. Natural childbirth enthusiasts believe that fear in labour slows the process and increases the chance of abnormal birth. In my experience, I have certainly noticed many women in strong labour at home, only for contractions to subside as they are transferred to hospital. Once they arrived labour would intensify again.

Antenatal education is not only for patients, it is also for midwives and doctors. There is much to learn. We assume that the major worry will be safety of the baby and fear of pain in childbirth.

> One woman agitated in her first pregnancy described her fear of vomiting being the only real worry. She felt confident in being able to manage the pain and was not fearful for the baby. In fact, the pregnancy and delivery went smoothly despite an extremely painful early labour. Only afterwards did I discover that my offer for pain relief was rejected not because she was coping with the pain but because she feared the drug would make her nauseous.

My education continued, and I learnt of the efficacy of using acupuncture to start labour. At the time I had thought it was unlikely to be of any use but later had to eat humble pie: three successive women due to be called for induction of labour were 'started off' by their friendly local acupuncturist. I know it does work sometimes, particularly if the neck of the womb is ripe and ready for labour. I now mention to mothers that some women have found acupuncture successful when they're faced with a date for admission to hospital to induce labour.

Recently, I was told of a study of pain in labour where the medical attendants graded the pain the women were suffering and then the women graded themselves. There was surprise as the two figures were wildly different. This reminds me not to make assumptions about what a person can or cannot bear. Equally chastening to me was a remarkable woman who had just delivered her first baby which had a cleft lip and palate, and who not only showed no revulsion or shock but was also determined to breastfeed and succeeded despite my negative mutterings.

Fear of Sick Children

P: 'Well, what's wrong with her, Doctor?'

D: 'As you can see I've had a really good look at her. She has a temperature and this fine rash you noticed. I'm sure she is suffering from a viral infection.'

P: 'What's it called?'

D: 'Well, I can't put a name to it, there are just so many different viruses.'

P: 'What treatment can you give her?'

D: 'I'm afraid antibiotics won't help with this sort of illness; all we can do is reduce the temperature by keeping her cool and giving her paracetamol.'

P: 'How do you know it's not meningitis? I read about that in the paper. They said children could have a fever and a rash – and some of them were dead in a few hours.'

D: 'I know it's all very frightening, but I can't find any sign of meningitis in your daughter.'

This interview hasn't gone very well for either doctor or patient. The patient knows the child is ill but this doctor can't put a name to it. The patient is confused, hearing worrying stories from the papers and possibly other parents. The doctor is unhappy as his professional competence is being threatened. The doctor is also concerned not to miss anything in the child who might eventually become ill with meningitis.

In earlier times it was easier: you could put a name to an unknown illness and then treat the child with a simple patent medicine. The parents' concern was satisfied: the doctor's professional integrity was intact.

Nowadays, parents and doctors are encouraged to face up to uncertainty: 'No, I can't say your child won't get meningitis. Yes, it is better to observe her carefully without treatment at the moment.'

The spin-off from such interactions should be a growing confidence in parents in coping with everyday childhood illnesses themselves. It should then follow that parents are in a position to pick up changes from the usual and to seek medical advice appropriately. The medical role switches to be a supporter of parental action and casts off the dependent patient situation.

Comments like: 'You know her much better than any doctors and are in the best position to observe' indicate recognition of the true situation and can be a support to parents.

Underlying parental fear of childhood illness are some of the instinctive feelings, of parenthood: deep love and fierce protectiveness. Some grandparents and parents cry openly, wishing to have the child's illness or disability themselves. The bond can surprise parents:

> One of my sons, as a two-year-old, walked backward towards the top of the stairs and then went down head-over-heels. Without even stopping to think I hurled myself head first down the stairs to save him. I spent 14 days limping and in pain whilst he was laughing at me groaning in a heap.

Watching your child breathless from asthma or having the chemotherapy injections for leukaemia is torture to any parent; adjusting to a diagnosis in your child is like a death. Parents go through all the stages of bereavement with initial disbelief and shock, to anger and rejection of advice, to wailing and grief and gradually to resolution and acceptance. In minor forms this process happens with every childhood illness and tests the doctor–parent relationship even if the process is understood.

Anger

In Chapter 1 I described how a patient and doctor might get to know one another. They might be able to work out a relationship based on mutual trust and understanding. Like most relationships, it doesn't always go right. The disagreements often come about when one party feels wronged and there is usually a confrontation.

In my experience these confrontations are of prime importance and are turning points in the relationship between doctor and patient. It is difficult to remember this when in the middle of an angry interchange, but on reflection it becomes clearer.

Some Causes for Anger

Inaccessibility

Many disputes revolve around accessibility. How available to his patients should a modern doctor be? Years ago the frightened relative may have been waiting outside the village church hoping the doctor might have time to call. Alternatively, the family of an ill patient might have walked miles to knock on the doctor's door in the middle of the night. More recently, before the advent of bleeps and mobile phones, the doctor could be contacted by telephone but remained out of contact whilst out on visits. Doctors' spouses were left to give advice for which they had not been trained. In inner cities doctors may have been out of contact even longer as public telephones were vandalized or patients too poor to have telephones.

In the event of a complaint about accessibility the terms and conditions of service for family doctors make it clear that they should be as available as would be expected by the average family doctor in their situation. Clearly, this average is constantly changing and may eventually require doctors to carry mobile phones as communication systems improve.

Getting the balance right is difficult. How can we protect ill patients from unavailable doctors and how can we protect doctors from unreasonable calls? In fact, the situation currently stands so that a family doctor may refuse to visit but must be able to account for, and be judged by, his decision not to visit.

One patient came with his wife to see me in the surgery. He had just been in hospital following a heart attack. He was in his early forties and had a pressurized job as a journalist. When he developed chest pain he put it down to indigestion but his wife persuaded him to go to hospital. In casualty he was seen and was quickly transferred to intensive care. He stayed in hospital 10 days and there had time to reflect on his life. He came to the surgery in the days after discharge from hospital.

Both the patient and his wife looked shattered and agitated. They seemed to expect a further attack at any time. We talked about the weeks ahead, the exercise, the return to work, the start of sexual activity. As we talked they pressed me for hard guidelines and exact details of each activity. When it came to what to do if he felt ill they wanted to know if they could speak to me. They wanted to have 24-hour access to their family doctor. I explained that this was not possible personally, but that we could offer 24-hour cover as a group of doctors. They became angry; it was clear they saw my attitude as hostile and saw me as a failure as a family doctor. I understood their feelings but thought of myself: no weekends away or no walks with the dogs in the country. They felt our service wasn't secure enough and wanted to know who would be at the end of the phone. They contacted a private doctor and arranged for his 24-hour cover.

Now, some years later, they have come back. The private doctor is gone and they no longer feel so anxious or isolated. The patient spends more time with his family and has decided never to work in the way he did. He starts the day with some exercise and values his leisure time. He also appreciates that my wish to have the same is reasonable and I think feels that my opinions are most likely to be balanced and sensible if I lead a balanced and sensible life. This row matured the relationship into a more meaningful one for patient and doctor.

Prejudice

The National Health Service was created to provide health care to all. Doctors are in a position to support or abuse this belief. In reality, they do both: on one hand they might visit favourite patients more often and generally take extra care of them, and at the same time crack down on patients who behave as if they expect more than their share of the service. Such hypocrisy should be avoided, of course, but it's a struggle.

One evening we were especially busy. I was doing a surgery for patients who felt ill that day (a non-appointment surgery). There were two left to be seen. One was Patrick, an old tramp who used to sing Irish ballads softly in the waiting room. His performances were discouraged but continued nevertheless fuelled by fortified lager. The second, an MP who was in a hurry to get to the House. Both had medical problems and Patrick was there first. At the time I thought my insistence to see them in order reflected a proper interpretation of the Health Service Act. The MP was furious and let me know it. I rigidly stuck to my principles. Later, on reflection, I realized my principles were based on prejudice. I was determined the MP should wait, particularly as his political beliefs ran contrary to mine. I imagined he would expect to be seen first, a figure in the community with an important job to do. I imagined he would prefer the destruction of the Health Service and all it stood for. In fact, the prejudice was all mine. Here he was, waiting his turn with his NHS GP. He had been prepared to put his beliefs on the line and fight for them. He was aware that Patrick would see another 15 minutes as further chance to be in the warm, assuming he had actually noticed at all. Fortunately, as family doctors, we get another chance to put things right and over the next couple of meetings we sorted it out, and I remember the row as an important learning experience for me.

Once, working as a GP in a small country town, I was aware of other examples of prejudice. The practice I worked in took all patients, but we heard rumours that some other practices in the town discouraged registration of Black and Asian families.

One elderly woman who used to visit me was a caricature of English village life: blue rinse, clipped hedges and Pekinese. She would talk about 'them' serving in the grocer's or moving in across the street. 'They' had too many children and 'their' food sent smells throughout the neighbourhood. She was, of course, an active member of her local church and was on the Parish Council.

My middle-class English upbringing and exposure to ladies like this somehow prevented a full-frontal attack. After all, she could have been my grandmother, who, having seen my Black best man kiss my wife-to-be, couldn't speak to me for a week. Eventually I found a way in after another of these outbursts. I expressed the notion that all people were God's children whatever their colour. She looked up sharply seeing she had been outflanked and took care never to broach the subject again with me.

Nowadays, I suspect I would be more confronting and be prepared to make my feelings more clear.

Another common situation is the prejudice between patients and 'foreign' doctors. One doctor I trained with repeated how often he had seen patients' faces fall as soon as they saw his black face. He would often get a surprised 'You speak English very well,' and he felt like replying, 'I ought to, you racist bastard, I was born here.' Certainly as a White doctor I often get remarks like, 'Oh, I saw a coloured doctor at the hospital. Actually [full of surprise], he/she was very nice.'

Apathy

'You just didn't care, when I rang up I told you she was ill and you told me you'd see her in the morning. It's too late now isn't it? Why couldn't you just get out of bed and come and see her? You just didn't care.'

This could be a doctor's nightmare, enough to wake him or her sweaty from sleep. And, of course, it could be true. The doctor may have lost the will to continue providing quality care. He or she may be ill or have personal problems that have affected clinical judgement. More commonly, the doctor may have considered the odds and made a blunder (see p. 104). Alternatively, the doctor may be thinking: 'That woman has called me out six times with chest pain over the last year and each time it's been nothing, it would be *this time* that I choose not to visit that she chooses to die.'

Apathy is a trait that most doctors would never hope to have. It runs contrary to all training and if adopted would signify professional suicide. Yet, it is an undeniable struggle at times: that last visit at night, the failure to check the dosage when tired, returning that last phone call . . .

Friday evenings and Sunday evenings are the times for 'The Absent Relative Syndrome'. This syndrome would be recognized by any family doctor. The telephone call might go something like this:

P: 'Oh, hello doctor, I'm sorry to ring you on Sunday night. I'm Mrs Thomas's daughter, you know Mrs Thomas of Newtown Road?'

D: 'Hello, yes I know her well, what's the problem?'

P: 'Well, my husband and I have been with mum this afternoon and she isn't as good as usual. Nothing particular, but her memory is poor. She had a cold last week she says, but she's over that. We wondered if you could pop in and see her tonight to check she's all right?'

D: 'What did you think I'd be able to do for her?'

P: 'Well, it's just that she might need help getting to bed and all that. We would stay but we both have jobs and need to be at work in the morning.'

D: 'Well, many people have got jobs to do in the morning and we would consider it your job to stay with mum if you are worried about how she will manage on a Sunday night.'

Thereafter the conversation will often deteriorate into a row. Similar calls are frequent; perhaps relatives are off to Spain for a month and want the doctor to call in their absence.

Insufficient respect

Both patients and doctors are aware of the respect that society gives doctors, and I have already described how this image can be the cause of embarrassment to both patient and doctor. It can also be the cause of angry confrontations.

> The widow of a titled industrialist would insist on ostentatiously using her title in the course of booking appointments at the surgery. Having fallen foul of using the wrong titles over the years I had long decided to avoid the whole issue and just use first and second names when calling in patients to be seen. She accused me of putting her down and deliberately shaming her in public. There followed a straight-talking session on both sides. I felt she saw why I avoided titles and I think I came to understand why it was important to her. She had worked hard behind the scenes to support her man who had risen fast in his business world. The initial money had been hers and he relied on her instinctive business acumen. When the knighthood came it was he that was in the limelight and she imagined years of retirement and reward for her efforts. In fact, he died leaving her less well provided for than she had hoped. I hoped that she felt understood and valued after our row, and she continued to visit even though she was never called by her title.

Such is the position that doctors are held in by society it is easily open to abuse. Every day doctors are flattered by courteous and respectful patients. Some of these attitudes may have been earned. In turn, doctors may show courtesy and respect for their patients. They may be proud of the work they do and have developed a realistic sense of value based on hard work, intensive training and self-assessment. They should believe in themselves and have the courage to say so.

Unfortunately, with daily bathings in society's adoration comes strutting self-importance from such reverence. The best cure for this is to become a patient oneself.

> One elderly practitioner was amazed to find he waited with patients in casualty. He shouted at the casualty doctors that he had been a family doctor for 30 years and that he wanted to be seen immediately. He was told to sit down and shut up. He was made to take his turn despite his protestations. He was full of

fear and pain and wanted help. He had till then lost the link between 'the patient' within himself and his patients.

Thereafter, he listened a little more carefully and felt his heart move a little more often.

Time

Time is a common focus for anger. Patients get angry for being kept waiting and doctors often refuse to see people who arrive late. 'Doctors just don't appreciate that people have other parts to their lives – we have jobs too and families to get to bed.' 'He kept me waiting for an hour last week and now isn't prepared to see me if I'm 10 minutes late.'

Time management is now a frequent subject for postgraduate study. These courses examine the factors which inhibit planning time well and those factors which assist. Some doctors function best on the principle that if a huge problem such as breast cancer or child abuse presents in the surgery it must be given time *then*. This time will have to be taken from others' booked appointments. It is hoped that those kept waiting will understand that they would get the same treatment should their need arise. Other doctors prefer a stricter time control, with patients asked to come back should a problem need more time.

It is certainly true that once the patient has been waiting more than 20 minutes the consultations get longer anyway. This is due to part of the time being taken for the doctor's apology and patients expressing anger or dissatisfaction or even understanding. In looking at the system one practitioner has varying appointment times chosen by the patient, who then is involved in time management. So the receptionist would say: 'How much time will you need with the doctor?' The patient may then choose either the two-minute, 10-minute or 12-minute slot. This is a nightmare to organize but suits some practices. As an experiment I tried to keep to time exactly, but it took enormous willpower, and I had a sense that I was creating work by not completing the tasks today. The patients clearly felt hassled and pushed, yet accepted that I might need to keep exactly to time. One or two who were busy efficient people were clearly delighted. I also had the feeling that the patients' response to knowing that only a 10-minute slot was available might encourage the problems to be disclosed earlier in the consultation. Psychotherapists insist that a session stops on the dot of 50 minutes even if an important issue has just been disclosed. Doctors might learn to do the same but it presents the doctor in a different light to patients. The traditional empathy, the caring, involved stance seems not in tune with today's time management skills.

I was infuriated by one patient who, despite repeated warnings, would always arrive late. I explained that his attitude was selfish and tried to get him to understand that with 3000 patients to look after the service wouldn't work his way. He looked bemused and I sensed he had a wider vision of time – he was floating through life without a care and I, anxious and stressed, was fighting to survive. I reassured myself that without 'my' attitudes the world would be inefficient and would have its progress halted. A doubt remained. This man was born and brought up in St Lucia, a small island in the eastern Caribbean. He had some serious medical problems that he was aware of, but had none of the neurotic frenzy that I would have had in his shoes. I felt in 'English' society he should assimilate and learn 'our' codes of behaviour.

I got the opportunity recently to travel with the family to the eastern Caribbean. We visited the Carnival in Trinidad and then, by boat and plane, saw eight different islands: it was a culture shock. Not only the beauty and the poverty, but more importantly the human qualities of the people. In particular, we felt the generosity: we were embarrassed to find our host had given up his house for us and slept downstairs on a sofa; relatives left work for the day to sit with us and show us round the islands. They gave time to us on a scale that was unheard of.

My St Lucia patient still arrives late. I understand why and have reflected on how ridiculous it all must seem through his eyes. I still give him a hard time, of course, but better understand his point of view.

Boundaries

A difficult area concerns the limits of the patient–doctor relationship. How much can we say to each other? What is acceptable behaviour? When do we feel the contact is intrusive and has got too close for comfort? When do we feel that the doctor has made assumptions about our attitudes and is acting on them?

Boundaries Checklist

1   Are you comfortable with this doctor?
2   Is it because of their dress, attitude, manner or beliefs? Do you trust their confidentiality? Do you trust your own feelings about them?
3   Which of the above do you want to be different?
4   Be prepared to explore and confront this issue, e.g. I feel uncomfortable talking about this as I am not sure how confidential our conversation is. e.g. I feel you have assumptions about me that are not correct. e.g. I think you are being over-familiar.
5   Following this discussion, do you still feel uncomfortable?
6   Consider changing your doctor.

Friendship

The advantage of having a doctor who really knows you often attracts friends to becoming patients. But it takes very little experience to show patients and doctors that this is usually a disaster. The friend back from a business trip with possible gonorrhoea requesting treatment and confidentiality is bad enough. But when he/she asks you to find an excuse to call his/her partner in for examination and treatment without ever knowing why, it shows how muddled it can get.

It is quite as bad for patients. How can you cope with your friend the doctor examining your piles, your genitals, discussing your sexual life or your marriage? Can you be angry and confrontational with the service you receive as a patient and not let this filter through into the friendship? In small, close-knit communities it is a fact of life that the doctor you saw and who examined you at 5 p.m. may be swimming next to you in the swimming pool or talking to you at dinner that same evening.

Who are these four people? The doctor and patient in the surgery and the doctor and patient at leisure. What thoughts do the four people have? 'I hope he's not going to mention I saw him/her at the surgery today'; 'Does he/she know I'm really off-duty now and I've got to have time for myself'; 'Now that my wife/husband/partner met his wife/husband/partner the other night, how can I come in to talk about my relationship?' 'Now that he has seen me shout at the kids how can he respect my advice about his?'

Both doctors and patients have anxieties about these difficult areas. Doctors who chat socially and mention issues raised in the confidential setting in the surgery soon lose their patients; patients who ring their medically qualified friends for advice out of hours soon stop being friends.

Most patients feel they want a doctor who they can complain to, agree with, get angry with, tell secrets to. They want him or her to be there if they are ill. They usually don't want to think about the distress or anxiety they might be causing in their friend the doctor when they are suffering themselves. Often this complex relationship does not work and the relationship has to change to be either friend or doctor.

Records

As a patient I am intrigued about what has been written in my medical notes. What did the doctor write about me as a child and what did he make of my parents? Unfortunately, I will never know as the records most probably are illegible and only mention the symptom and the treatment given.

Many patients feel the records are theirs and that they must be available to be read; many doctors feel the records are really theirs and *no way* will patients read them. In fact, technically, the records belong to the Minister of Health and with current legislation neither can claim ownership. Recent changes in the law allow patients to see records made from 1st November 1991.

The most useful records for doctors are usually those that not only record facts but also record impressions and ideas. Would the next doctor faced with an ill child find record A or B more helpful:

A   Fever 3 days, no contacts/travel.
     On examination no signs, temp. 37.8 P.90
     ? Viral infection
     Fluids and paracetamol
B   Fever 3 days, came in with mother 7 p.m.
     sister and family well
     Full examination, no cause found, temp. 37.8 P.90
     Mother rarely consults – worried by the look of him *Watch*
     See tomorrow if not better
     ?check urine ?full blood test ?paediatric referral
     Mentioned to partner on call

or what about C or D for an older patient?

C   Tired, no energy, 3 months
     No relation to anything else
     On examination no cause found
     Full blood count, see one week
D   Tired 3 months, can't see why but 'I feel half dead'
     Last felt like this 10 years ago and can't see why
     Job: Fashion buyer, no change
     Relationship: Steve 2 years 'OK'
     Sister: 'Successful job earns twice as much as her'
     Parents: Father died 1980 leukaemia
     Mother alive and well
     On examination nil found
     For FBC to rule out anaemia (and leukaemia) and so we can talk next week ?Unresolved grief ?Conflict with sister
     For further talk.

The patient may feel that doctors have no right to record subjective impressions. After all, what chance do patients have to note: 'Saw Dr . . . today seemed more interested in my Dad with his leukaemia than with why I'm so tired'?

On balance it would be best if impressions were explored in

the consultation so as to establish fact. However, such exploration takes time and the success of subsequent visits often depends on the doctor and patient continuing where they left off. Notes in the style of A and C leave the doctor with few memory cues and have no flavour. Notes in the style of B and D prepare for the next meeting with ideas and action.

For patients facing doctors holding their records, the following may give an idea of how to explore the sorts of records the doctor is making:

P:　'Doctor, do you record everything I say to you?'

D:　'What would you not want me to record?'

P:　'Well, supposing I wanted to talk to you about a secret in the family or something I was ashamed of years ago?'

Imagine three possible replies to this question:

D:　(i)　'I am happy not to record specific incidents in the notes that you are worried about.'

(ii)　'It is my decision what I record in the notes so don't tell me anything you might not want in your records?'

(iii)　'I find that question difficult to answer as there are some situations that involve other people's health and safety, or your health and safety, that I must record, but I won't know if what you are about to say is one of those situations.'

In all three possible answers the patient is now in the position to judge what he or she can safely say. The patient has also gained an insight into her doctor which may or not help her to achieve trust.

Gifts

Doctors generally enjoy the respect of society, trust of their patients and a satisfactory income. Some have chosen medicine in the hope they 'do good'. This honourable aim carries the risk that doctors might *need* to be respected and thanked for the work they do. We all need thanks and support but do doctors need it more?

Patients sometimes thank their doctors with gifts. Gifts are often from those who can least afford it or who have followed the most straightforward diagnosis and treatment:

> . . . two fillet steaks one morning on the surgery desk, a gift from the village butcher (he had lifted a side of beef and damaged his back the night before and had needed an injection for pain, then had managed to go to work and was grateful); the plastic bag full of half-used tubes of skin ointment, boxes of plasters and old bandages given by a mentally ill woman who thought they could be put to good use; the fine bottles of wine from grateful parents following memorable births; the boxes of chocolates for my children for caring for elderly spinsters.

These gifts are all special and doctors are especially fortunate to receive them. Churlish though it may seem, sometimes, however, the gifts are more complicated than a simple thank you. They may mean 'You haven't forgotten me have you?' 'Will you come to my home if I get ill this year?' 'You won't nag me about my smoking when I come to the surgery next week?' These complicated gifts need to be made simple. The doctor must obviously thank the patient but also re-establish boundaries, leaving the patient in no doubt about business returning to normal, whether that's about smoking or a confrontation about other health issues.

Family

Some readers have a doctor in the family and some will have found no difficulty in 'boundaries' with this relationship. Others, however, will have noticed that doctors often make unsound judgements when emotionally involved with their patients. Senior surgeons miss appendices in their own children; skin doctors tend to think of rare and dangerous causes to simple uncomplicated rashes; GPs tend to neglect their spouses' and children's health, and there is often little room to be ill in the doctor's house.

All night I worried about the simple advice I gave to a sick member of my own family – advice which I could have given to one of my other patients without a second thought. But with this 'patient' the implication of getting it wrong was too much to handle comfortably and it was a great relief to hand the problem over to their usual GP in the morning.

Talking to a travel agent friend she says that family holidays booked through her always seem to go wrong and cause much distress, and I realize this affects most walks of life.

Doctors' families deserve the best medical care and that means their own doctor who knows where his/her boundaries are.

Confidentiality

Some consultations start with 'I don't know whether I should tell you what I'm going to say' or with 'I am too ashamed/ embarrassed to talk about . . . If you can promise me never ever to talk about this to anyone . . .'

As doctors we might feel that the moment of revelation of a deep family secret is imminent. However, alarm bells should ring for doctors and patients at this moment. The next stage of the consultation might reveal a murderer, a child at risk or a patient with a serious transmissible disease.

A family secret was so deep and well protected that it had caused a serious emotional disturbance in the family, and particularly the daughter. She was violent and prone to self-mutilation – it seemed she sensed a missing link. Protecting the parents' secret seemed cruel in view of their daughter's confusion and distress. But to reveal it might cause immediate danger to another person. I imagined she might even want to kill her parents.

The revelation of sexually transmitted diseases and now human immunodeficiency virus (HIV) and AIDS in families carry the particular need for confidentiality, but what if this confidentiality puts another person's life at risk?

Many doctors believe that they have little responsibility to inform parents of their young teenager's request for contraception. Most would agree that they would try to counsel the patient to discuss this sensibly with their parents. Others believe that 'children' under 16 should have few confidentiality rights and that parents should be informed. It is likely that neither patients nor doctors will agree on these issues.

For patients the dilemma is complicated by not knowing where the confidentiality boundaries lie. In what circumstances will confidentiality not be protected? Patients must ask doctors in what situations they disclose information, and doctors must try to explain their boundaries to patients.

For example:

'What is your attitude to disclosing medical information to insurance companies? Do you describe my life-style and habits and relationships?'

'What would you tell my social worker if she/he rang for information?'

'What would you say to my parents if I talk to you about my worries?'

An adolescent boy behaved in a way that made me worry for his safety. He described feelings of self-hate and indifference to over-use of the family's pain-killers. I felt my concern fo. him over-ruled his rights for confidentiality. I rang his parents and asked them to come in with him. Even though I sensed his pleasure that his parents now knew about it, he decided to find another doctor for himself who wouldn't contact his parents in future. Was I right or should I have held on to this potentially dangerous situation and risked an overdose in order to protect the trust of the relationship which has now gone?

These confidentiality issues are difficult and need careful counselling of the patient and often support for the doctor from his/her colleagues.

What is allowed? Can there be agreement on what is acceptable to patients and doctors?

Dress

Do patients get upset by doctors without ties or without white coats? Do doctors get upset by patients who dress outrageously?

I can think of respected, conscientious and kind doctors who have been both the tie-less and white-coat variety. Indeed, I have known GPs do surgeries in shorts and tee-shirts, dressing gown and slippers and even in three-piece suits and buttonhole. Similarly, I can think of some patients who always wear six layers of clothing or who never wash or who wear underwear with a provocative message on it, or who refuse to take their clothes off, or who take any excuse to remove them.

There may be signals from either patient or doctor that can be followed. Is there evidence of tolerance of both sides? Would a punk rocker be prepared to see a doctor in a suit or would he or she assume that there could be no dialogue? Would a doctor be prepared to thoroughly examine someone who was mentally ill and who was unaware of his offensive smell? Doctors and patients must be sensitive to signals from each other; both must be prepared to protect their own boundaries. A patient can say that he is ill at ease with a doctor in a white coat or that he feels uncomfortable with a doctor in jeans and trainers. Similarly, doctors should be able to ask patients to be considerate in the surgery in their dress. To change from muddy boots or oily overalls and, if necessary, to ask uninhibited patients to be more discreet. The key to a successful working relationship is this mutual respect, and boundaries are part of it.

Time

Patient says:

'I won't keep you a tick doctor, you've got a full surgery out there.'

Doctor thinks:

'You always get in and out quickly and never talk about how hard it is to manage with all your problems. How have you always got time for everybody?'

or perhaps

'You always say that and do stay 30 minutes and always make me late'.

Doctor says:

'Sorry to keep you waiting so long, we've been very busy.'

Patient thinks:

'Heavens! Don't you think we are busy too? I rushed from work to get here for an *appointment* and I was kept for an *hour*!'

or perhaps

'I know you've been talking to that Mrs . . . who lost her husband last week. I really don't mind, it could have been me.'

These thoughts are often expressed by both patients and doctors. Such a dialogue often releases the tension under the surface. Increasingly pressure of time seems to be part of our daily lives.

Patients and doctors can together manage time better. First, appointment systems can be designed to allow consultations at convenient times for doctors and patients.

Secondly, patients can ask doctors: 'How much time can you give me to discuss this today?' or 'When can I arrange to speak to you further about this problem?' Doctors can also say: 'I am afraid I can only give you 10 minutes today. Please come back on . . .' or 'We have discussed this for 15 minutes today, and I can't see any progress. Let's meet again next week.' This 'kicking for touch' is usually acceptable to patients and doctors. Both are saying that they want future contact but that there is a time limit to the contact today.

Behaviour

Codes of behaviour vary from surgery to surgery and from town to town. I know well-loved doctors who have thrown patients out of their waiting room at 6 p.m. saying 'My opinion's not worth having after 6 p.m. – come back in the morning.' Others refuse to see smokers and would never see a patient with alcohol on his or her breath. At the other extreme are doctors who smoke and drink in company with patients. These examples are from either end of a wide spectrum of behaviour.

Patients' behaviour is no less diverse. From the self-effacing 'I don't believe in troubling you unless I was dying' to banging the desk and 'demanding my rights'. It is easy to remember the extremes: the sad, quiet man who stole his records from reception and then burnt them in the toilet; the elderly woman who attacked me with her umbrella because she believed I had stopped her home help. Once again each doctor and each patient must examine each other's behaviour boundaries for the relationship to be fruitful.

Space

Space, like time, is a cause for conflict and concern between doctors and patients. Some doctors think it is a luxury not to have patients as neighbours. This is, of course, only usually possible in London as city living allows the doctor to live close to the surgery but outside the practice area. Here, neighbours can just be neighbours and friends be friends.

The country has many attractions, and village life, with the complex friend/doctor relationship poses few problems to most. I feel this relationship will only work with deep trust and understanding of boundaries on both sides.

Knowing the doctor lives down the lane is a comfort to a family with a collapsed relative or following a road traffic accident. I think most doctors see that as an occupational hazard – something that goes with the job – but what about 'Auntie's visiting from abroad and has run out of her heart pills' or 'Do you mind quickly checking Johnny's ear as I don't want to call the doctor out.'

Each doctor and patient has his own idea of what's reasonable. It is possible to discover where those ideas clash before the event occurs.

Another 'space' issue comes up in the surgery. The patient is usually shown a chair that suits the doctor's consulting style. It may be across the corner of a desk or alongside or directly opposite; indeed, there may be no desk at all. But what about the patient? Some patients move the chair away from the desk, or nearer to the doctor, making their statement about where they feel comfortable and asserting individuality. We may inadvertently invade each other's space with touch or closeness and should be prepared to state if this is happening. Picking up non-verbal signs of this is discussed in the next section on language.

Language

Body Language

Body language is part of every human contact. Unwittingly, we are all experts at using it. In a room full of people we know who is attracted to us, and who is hostile. By a complex exchange of non-verbal cues we pass messages to one another. It is possible with training and experience to heighten awareness of body language and to use it constructively in the consultation between doctor and patient. Many young family doctors will have been trained to observe for the cues of inner distress and unspoken emotion. The restless feet of the uncomfortable patient who is keen to leave. The crossed arms and legs of the defensive patient who feels exposed. The removing and restoring of the wedding ring in someone talking about their marriage. It is not necessary to point out these signs to the patient, but merely to use the information that is there to see:

> 'I sense you find it embarrassing talking about this subject.'

> 'I feel you are angry with me.'

> 'I suspect part of you wants to leave your marriage and part wants to stay.'

For those who feel this is too big a step to take, then a prefix of 'Please tell me if I've got this completely wrong, but I feel . . .' could be used.

It often comes as a complete surprise to the patient that their feelings can be observed, especially when the body behaviour is contrary to what is being said. Surprise can also be felt by the doctor. When consulting, the doctor is often deep in concentration: thinking about possible diagnoses, assessing influences on the patient, symptoms and being alert to body language. It sometimes feels as if one is behind a one-way mirror, heard but unobserved. Frequently this feeling is shattered by the perceptive patient:

'Am I boring you, doctor?'

'You look as if you are in a hurry, doctor.'

'Are you all right, doctor? Should I come back another time?'

Knowing about body language sometimes seems to help.

Seeing the patient mirror one's own body language is a sign of concentration and effective communication. If one leans on one elbow the patient will lean as if copying you in the mirror. Move to another posture and the patient will follow. Being too conscious of these changes can detract from the natural flow of communication and be a distraction.

Some years ago I went to hear an expert on body language. He spoke persuasively about the cultural differences in non-verbal communication. Amongst many examples of ethnic variation he believed that Black Afro-Caribbeans communicate with more whole body movement and less eye-to-eye contact. To white northern Europeans this body language might appear restless and shifty. He also explained that the more static posture with a greater degree of eye-to-eye contact would appear rigid and threatening to some Blacks. I could see how such differences could enhance misunderstanding. In the surgery, as with all of us, Black patients can feel nervous and exposed. As a doctor trained in body language, would my attempts to use more whole body language with less eye contact be received as 'Here's a doctor I can talk to' or, more likely, 'What's the matter with this doctor who's moving all over the place and won't look at me?'

Perhaps the answer is to be oneself, but to understand and respect cultural differences. The body language of this understanding and respect will be seen by patients just as clearly as any prejudice or hostility the doctor may hope to hide.

Jargon

As with most professionals, doctors love jargon; it comforts them and supports the magic and mystery of medicine. I still enjoy the sound of 'Osgood–Schlattor's Disease' or 'De Quervains Tenosynovitis'. Occasionally, the patient shares the delight and carries the name like a medal on show. I suspect the most common response is a yawn and a sense of being excluded from what's actually going on. Some patients correctly comment that: 'You may be feeling better now you've put a long name on it, but what does the illness mean to me?'

Medical language means different things to different people. Peter, a surgeon, is particularly careful not to use jargon when talking to patients.

> Peter sat down on the patient's bed in hospital and explained the piece (biopsy) of bowel (colon) removed for further tests (histological analysis) did, unfortunately, show cancer (carcinoma). A major operation (colonectomy) would be needed to remove it. The patient listened carefully and seemed to understand. He checked whether she had anything to ask and was surprised by the reply 'No doctor. I understand. Anyway, thank God it's not cholecystitis.' How could he start to tell this woman that cholecystitis is a gall bladder infection easily treated these days? The operation he planned was going to remove half her large bowel and he might find evidence of cancerous spread to other organs. How could she compare an infection with what might be her final illness? In shock, Peter asked, 'Cholecystitis?' The patient then explained how her mother had died in agony. Her cholecystitis had led to peritonitis and it was only discovered after death at the post-mortem examination. It was a good example of how patients and doctors need to work together to make sure they understand each other.

I remember one uncomfortable occasion when I was unable to understand the patient's 'jargon'.

A fit-looking man in his fifties had come in for a check-up. He had been found to have high blood pressure at a work medical. Indeed, on checking it I realized he was going to need some treatment for it, and I told him so. He answered that he thought his blood pressure would always be up when he had 'love balls'. I obviously looked blankly at him, 'Love balls?' He went on, 'You know, doc, when you haven't had a woman for a while and you get that terrible aching in your balls.' At this point I came clean and announced I had never had this condition. He looked amazed. I could see his opinion of me shrinking by the second. I almost wished I could have this dreadful pain. He tried harder to describe the feeling in fuller and fuller detail, determined that I should recognize it. I rather weakly murmured, 'Perhaps I've just been lucky,' and changed the subject.

Jargon is not only the protector of professionalism and maintainer of the magic; it is also to save us embarrassment. Doctors have constructed a complicated way to communicate about bodily functions when simple ways already existed. We believe that patients defaecate, urinate, expectorate and ejaculate. In fact, different patients use different words, and we need only to ask to find out what they are. This medical language may not only alienate the patient, but may obscure meaning to the point where communication is lost. Using the patients' own words for things is simpler and shows respect for them and their codes of belief. It tends to lower tension, after all, if the doctor can say those words without embarrassment and then the patient may feel more able to talk.

Accents and Cultural Language

As a medical student working on a building site in the holidays, I had a boss who was a large Cockney carpenter. He shouted barely understood orders from the top of the ladder and I would scuttle up and down bringing what he needed. One of these orders was for 'French' nails. Some minutes later, after I had searched all the boxes, he descended. With much abuse of my common sense, despite so much education, he showed me the box of three-inch nails.

Faced with patients who don't understand, I remember his irritation. I try to remember to write things down or draw pictures and diagrams to make requests or information clearer. Often the patient is pleased to bring an interpreter – they can be vital, but sometimes not.

A Russian couple, childless after 10 years, came to talk about the wife's stomach pain. This pain was growing, it started 10 years ago and was now 'violent'. The husband struggled with the English–Russian Dictionary. I asked for an interpreter at our next meeting and the husband looked shattered: 'I can speak English.' I wondered how to explain through his proud, but limited English, that the pain was grief. She had had many exploratory operations and investigations to determine why she hadn't got pregnant. I wanted to explain that they might have to accept that they might not conceive and that the pain of this thought could cause a growing ache in her stomach. It was also clear that to ask for someone else to interpret for her seemed a rejection of him, a man who already carried an enormous sense of failure.

Failing to understand the doctor is just as common. Regional accents and GPs born abroad (now 23 per cent of total number of GPs) mean that the doctor may be misunderstood. It is not good enough for the patient to feel the doctor was very kind but was unable to understand a word. The patient must complain and the foreign doctor must not see this as necessarily racist. After all, good communication is the heart and soul of the patient–doctor relationship, and the doctor must get further training in language if needed. But it is not always easy when the doctor is born and bred in the UK. The patient may feel 'peeliwally' (Scots for lethargic) or a bit 'queer' or 'bilious' if an elderly patient. Some patients talk of being 'below par' or 'under the weather' and it is difficult to see how 'foreign' doctors can make sense of these expressions.

Who's in Charge?

This area of difficulty is part of nearly every consultation in general practice. Patient and doctor frequently jockey for control of the consultation and often settle for a compromise on the cause of the illness, the actual diagnosis and the suitable treatment. In Chapter 1 (see p. 16) this 'jockeying' is described in the first meeting with the doctor. Here in this section I want to look at the issue of who's in charge in particular situations that often lead to difficulties.

Diagnosis

It would seem obvious that the doctor is in charge of diagnosis; after all, it's the patient who apparently has come in to ask for professional judgement and advice. In fact, this is often far from the case, and it is in the interests of all doctors and patients for it not to be the case.

> An isolated single man came in to get his certificate. He had been certified as unfit for work many years ago. He suffered with arthritis and in reality had never recovered fully from a nervous breakdown in wartime. As was so common then, the cause of his disability was stated as a vague muscular and rheumatic disorder to protect the doctors and patient from facing the painful issues. I sensed that he saw himself as a failure in society's eyes and had isolated himself from life as a result. He felt persecuted and was suspicious of even well-meaning neighbours. In the course of collecting his certificate he mentioned that he had a painful rash around his chest. He wondered if anything could help it. As I examined him he stated that he knew the cause of it was from being pricked by a holly tree that he had cut down the week before.
>
> In fact, he had a classic case of shingles. I started the negotiating with, 'I am doubtful that a holly bush could cause a rash like this, I think it's shingles.' He responded with, 'Oh no doctor, it's the holly bush that scratched me. It's exactly the same spot.' With another patient I might have explained why I was so sure. How the pain would have come before the shingles rash, and surely he had noticed it made him feel tired and low, as shingles does. I might have explained what an extraordinary illness shingles is, how the chicken pox virus, after emerging as a common children's illness, will lodge itself in a nerve only to

return decades later. What a feat of survival, I would have
warned him that contact with the shingles rash can spread
chicken pox but not another attack of shingles . . .

But I didn't. Initially, I felt angry and put down. How could he
be so stupid not to realize he was wrong. For a moment I
thought he could just put up with his 'holly-bush rash' with no
help from me. After this burst of internal anger I remembered he
was a sad, isolated man who must have made others feel like I
do. After all, what has he got? Why should I try to take his idea
away from him? After all, the shingles would get better anyway,
and he wouldn't be in contact with anyone. I explained that I
thought the rash would get better on its own and suggested
some pain-killers. He, of course, refused; grown men didn't need
pain-killers for a holly-bush rash.

In this consultation the patient was firmly in control of the
diagnosis. Confronting the patient, which I would normally
advocate, would have been destructive in his case.

Usually the 'jockeying' is more subtle and is very much
dependent on the consultation skills of the doctor.

A patient, an overweight 45-year-old man, complains of low back
pain. After listening to the story and examining the patient the
doctor feels that this is simple muscular strain caused by poor
posture and obesity. If the doctor takes charge and states his
idea, the patient may agree and set course for a future life of
fitness. He may, of course, ignore this opinion and continue as
he is.

Somehow the doctor has to help the patient to explain what the
backache means to him. Some starting lines might be:

   (i)   'Why do you think this backache has come?'
   (ii) 'What made you come with this backache?'
   (iii) 'Who else has backache in your family and contacts?'
   (iv) 'How do you think we can get this better?'

From these open questions may come the answers that explain
the diagnosis. Two potential answers from each question:

(i) 'I think the backache came because I lifted some paving
     stones at the weekend – and I'm not as young or fit as I
     was.'
     'I think the backache came because I get it whenever I'm
     tense – it's been hell at work recently.'

(ii) 'Oh, I came because I can't work with this, I'll need a
     certificate.'
     'I came because I was worried about a disc. My dad had
     disc trouble and had to have an operation.'

(iii) 'Well, it's got nothing to do with it, but a mate at work has
     just been told he's got bone cancer – I couldn't have that
     could I?'
     'No one actually. My family has always had strong backs –
     I can't understand it. Why do you think I've had this
     trouble?'

(iv) 'I just hoped it was nothing serious. I'll manage with pain-
     killers if it's only a muscle strain.'
     'That's what I came to see you for doctor. I'll be happy to
     try anything to get rid of the pain.'

From each open question could come a number of answers that
allow the doctor to see the range of the patient's experience,
belief and attitude to the problem. The more open the question
the better. In fact:

'What do you think of this?'
'What do you know about backache?'
'How does it make you feel?'

are even more likely to get at the patient's view of his illness.
Without this perspective the doctor's diagnosis and treatment
may run contrary to belief and understanding, and will therefore not be effective.

Both patient and doctor can be in control of which questions
to ask and which answers to give. Both may withhold their
feelings if not in tune with each other. In many successful
consultations the final result is likely to be a compromise;
the diagnosis may be one that the patient and the doctor can
accept.

Treatment

Who's in charge?

The popular model does sometimes happen:

The patient feels ill and goes to the doctor

The doctor diagnoses the complaint and recommends treatment

The patient accepts diagnosis and treatment

Both are happy
(secure in role)

This model happens every day across the country. Pills are swallowed, injections are given, creams applied and suppositories inserted.

The model only works if there is trust in the relationship as described in Chapter 1 (see p. 22). Power can then be safely shifted to doctor or to patient, depending on the situation.

Situation 1: Power shift to patient
Mrs Elderfield, a retired dance teacher, comes to the surgery with a breast lump. She only recently 'noticed it' despite its hard nature and large size. In fact, the skin is stretched over it and is glossy. She explains that she was going to leave it but she knows her daughter would be upset if she hadn't discussed it with the doctor. The doctor examines the patient, notices the hard, fixed swelling tethered to the skin and knows it's cancer:

D: 'Well, Mrs Enderfield, do you know what this is?'

P: 'It's cancer isn't it doctor?'

D: 'Yes it is.'

P: 'It doesn't hurt at all, you know doctor.'

D: 'Cancers in the breast *are* usually painless, but you must be upset about it.'

P: 'Well, the idea isn't nice is it? But we all have to get something. What will happen doctor?'

D: 'I'm sorry, I'm not clear what you are asking me.'

P: 'Well, I'm 83 now. How long do you think I've got?'

D: 'I'm afraid I can't tell you that, and of course it may depend on what treatment is given.'

P: 'Oh, I wouldn't want any treatment.'

D: 'Sometimes surgery is not necessary and it just means some tablets and X-ray treatment.'

P: 'No, I wouldn't want that.'

D: 'Would you prefer to come back after giving it all some thought and bring your daughter with you so we can discuss it in greater depth?'

P: 'It's kind of you doctor, but I've made up my mind. I'm not having anything done to it and my daughter knows I wouldn't. I have never been to hospital in my life and I don't want to start that now.'

D: 'How did you get to feel like that about hospitals and medicines?'

P: 'I watched my brother go through it all and he had no part of himself left at the end.'

D: 'That sounds awful – were you very close?'

P: 'Yes, but it's a long time ago and I've got over it. I just wouldn't allow the same to happen to me.'

D: 'All right, but I feel I ought to warn you what might happen if you don't have some treatment.'

P: 'All right doctor.'

D: 'Well, with the lump being the size it is, the skin is tight and it's likely the skin will get thinner and the cancer will grow through the skin. When this happens you would need regular dressings and many patients get upset by the thought and look of it.'

P: 'I understand that, but it's better that way.'

D: 'I just must be quite clear you understand that in other women cancers often don't spread and kill you. They can frequently be completely cured by modern treatments even when they have grown as yours has. By deciding as you have, it may be you are embarking on years of dressings and discomfort when this is not necessary.'

P: 'I understand what you are saying, but I won't change my attitude about it.'

D: 'All right, I can see you have made your mind up. If you change your mind or want to discuss it further please let me know. In any case, we would be pleased to help with dressings or other treatments should you want it.'

P: 'Thank you doctor. I'll call you if I need you.'

The patient stayed firm. In fact, she did not call anyone until six months later. Then she asked for help with dressings. She had been buying gauze squares and it was getting too expensive for her; the chemist suggested she might get them free on prescription. The cancer had come through the skin and weeped fluid and had begun to smell. The nurses helped her to dress it and showed her how to use the effective sprays that disguise the smell. She wouldn't let anyone touch it and I continued to see her out shopping and chatting to friends in the street. No one else ever knew. When she did die, it was following a fall and a fractured hip. She was taken to hospital despite protests and operated on to fix the hip. She died in the days that followed. She had had some years at home carrying on as before, until this accident. I was not surprised that she had died once she had gone to hospital for the first time in her life.

The patient in the story stayed in charge throughout. The doctor tried repeatedly to take control but was foiled. The doctor's anxiety revolved around the idea that perhaps he had not made it clear enough or perhaps he had said something that had put her off. With experience it becomes easier to accept the patient taking charge and only looking for ways to assist them in their decision.

Situation 2 – Power shift to doctor

Being in charge and being given permission to take control is something we may all want from our doctors when we're ill. I would hope I will be able to tell my doctor to take over, particularly in situations such as surgical emergencies and heart attacks.

With mental health issues it is often different. The responsibility may be with the doctor and the power will have come from the Mental Health Act. The patient may be fighting to keep control of his diagnosis and his treatment, but the doctor may have to judge if the patient's mental state puts himself or others at risk. Often there is this nightmare time in mental breakdowns when the patient's behaviour is worsening, his or her insight diminishing, and the risk to him or herself is slowly increasing. At this time there may be insufficient evidence of risk to force admission to hospital under a 'Section' (Mental Health Act Sections).

One such patient, a secretary to a firm of solicitors, was noticed to have been behaving strangely. Initially, it had been odd remarks at work. These remarks had been of a religious nature, recommending clients to seek help from their spiritual adviser rather than the legal profession.

When her disturbance became worse the solicitors suggested she sought medical help, but she refused politely. Eventually, her job was on the line, she accepted and came to see me. In the consultation I was struck by the vitality of this young woman who claimed to have had a religious conversion. She had decided to seek admission to a convent and eventually to take Holy Orders. She explained how so many of the clients at her work had lost their way in the world, and she increasingly felt it her duty to guide them to truth. I was concerned that she seemed to have few social contacts and had alienated members of her family. I was also concerned by her preoccupation with the 'bread' and 'the body of Jesus Christ'. At this stage there were no overt signs of madness and she refused any help. Later that week her mother rang to say that she thought her daughter was having a 'breakdown' and that I had to do something. She felt there had been a complete character change and she knew something was wrong. I apologized and explained I could not discuss any patient's case with a relative, and would need written permission from the patient to do so. The mother was furious and rang off. The patient then lost her job. She had suddenly raged at a client and the partners felt that they could not keep her any longer. There followed increasing numbers of calls from neighbours claiming strange behaviour at her home. I called repeatedly but she was always out.

Eventually a priest telephoned me to explain that she had undressed completely in her local church and had been taken into custody by police. From there she was transferred to the local mental hospital. I was asked to come and assess her with a view to a Section 2, a compulsory one month's assessment order in hospital.

The patient I saw there had deteriorated. She believed she was at one with Jesus Christ, that their bodies could be joined in perpetuity. She knew she had the spirit inside her and could hear voices that instructed her what to do. She was agitated and believed everyday objects with her had a special religious significance and this was a sign from God.

When I explained that I was about to sign papers to enforce her assessment in hospital, she became angry and abusive. She refused to stay and said that I had no power to do this.

Many months later, back in the bosom of the family, she was a broken reed, the vitality gone. Looking back she understood some of what had happened and remembered it all. She apologized for her behaviour and I expressed the wish that we could have been more successful in getting her help sooner. She expressed no resentment for her treatment and my part in it. I wondered how she would ever recover fully from the incident and wished somehow it was possible to protect freedom of the individual yet avoid situations like this.

Alternatives

Being 'in charge' can certainly be uncomfortable, but doctors can get very upset about alternatives. Any of these three situations could be a cause for 'difficulties':

(i)   'Oh doctor, could you give me some of these tablets? My homeopath says I can get them on the National Health.

(ii) 'I've seen a specialist in Harley Street who has found out the cause of my problems. I have an overgrowth of yeasts in my bowel. He tells me I can get you to have a special test to prove it.'

(iii) 'I have stopped the blood pressure tablets. My naturopath says that I won't need them now that I'm on this special diet.'

The common factor in all these situations is a conflict over 'who's in charge'. The patient is bringing to one professional the views of another. It may be that the family doctor is felt to be unapproachable and the patient is punishing him with a good doctor or alternative practitioner. It may be that the alternative practitioner or specialist is keen to keep the family doctor as the bad doctor and colludes with the patient. Together they arrange treatments without proper communication in writing. It may also be that the family doctor has failed to listen to the patient's needs and has alientated them.

Disputes over control and attitudes are common. Doctors tend to speak as if they own their patients who, like children, need to be kept under control. They become hurt when the patients turn to other 'parents'. Of course, the relationship works best when the power stays with the patient and the professionals become independent advisers.

Instead of getting angry with the patient wanting homeopathic pills, the doctor could, appropriately, be angry at the failure of proper communication from another colleague. Instead of getting angry at the idea of a special test for this cure of all complaints, the family doctor should be requesting a written explanation of the special test. Similarly, the diet could be given a go should the professionals agree to test it with the co-operation of the patient.

If the original contract between patient and family doctor has been negotiated satisfactorily then disputes of who's in charge are minimal. The contract may need re-shaping as time goes on, but that is part of healthy exchange as doctor and patient respond to their changing world.

Referrals and Second Opinions

Patients get referred for many reasons. At the simplest level it may be that the doctor and patient have identified a problem that needs further treatment: the painful neck that would benefit from physiotherapy or the inflamed appendix that needs the surgeon's knife. Even at this 'simple' level there can be problems: the physiotherapy may not be available immediately, and the doctor is expected to shop around to find the quickest service for their patients; the patient may be unhappy to face surgery at a particular hospital as it may be full of painful memories of a relative's death.

Patients may also be referred on because the doctor does not know what is wrong: the strange rash that does not fit into the common patterns encountered in family practice; the cause of falls in an elderly patient.

Problems arise here too as the patient often feels the doctor is not being straightforward with him/her and is disguising his fear of a more serious illness. This may be true and the doctor is keen not to talk to the patient about something that has only a small risk of being correct.

Patients may also request a second opinion or even third opinion. These are difficult to ask for as patients know they can be destructive of the patient–doctor relationship. If the doctor has diagnosed a complaint and treatment is underway the doctor may feel threatened by the patient's request for a second opinion. Sometimes the patient has had the opinion of many doctors, yet still wants more, perhaps wanting a second diagnosis rather than a second opinion. Of course, the patient may have heard of somebody who, only after years of trying, found a doctor who understood or revealed the true cause of what ailed him or her.

Second opinions are also problematic as getting an independent second opinion can be difficult. The letter sent to the specialist may say 'Thank you for seeing this man with chest pain and palpitations'. It also may say 'Than!: you for seeing this man who consults us day and night and is sure he is dying from heart disease. I think his chest pain is muscular and palpitations just anxiety.'

The first letter is factual and may prevent the specialist having an insight into how the patient behaves in general practice. The second letter is impressionistic and may prevent the patient getting a fair assessment. In practice, these problems rarely cause serious difficulties as doctors are usually keen to find the diagnosis that has been missed by colleagues over the years. The reply from the specialist might say 'Thank you for sending Mr P. along today. His chest pain and palpitations are due to . . . and although rare in a man of his age must never be forgotten.'

Patients are often surprised to find that they need a family doctor's letter to get a second opinion at all, especially if they have decided to pay for this opinion. The roots of this ruling are sensible. The second opinion should be informed of past medical history and drug allergies perhaps forgotten by the patient. They should also be informed of current treatment prescribed and have access to the opinions and investigations performed by other specialists.

Often the request for a family doctor's letter is seen by the patient as part of the 'doctors' club'. The 'club' keeps power in the profession and prevents the patient getting an honest and independent appraisal. The 'club' might also be seen as a way to keep relationships between doctors sweet and cosy and leave the way clear for more private referrals for second opinions in future.

The truth in these situations can only be sorted out in the surgery where the limits of trust are negotiated and established. My impression over the years is that the relationship with the patient is rarely, if ever, sacrificed at the expense of the 'doctors' club'.

Finally, the referral to another agency might be to buy time or space from each other. The patient may be consulting frequently and the doctor and patient can be locked in a pattern that they are unable to break. Perhaps the patient is repeatedly asking for help with a variety of symptoms. Each symptom is looked at in detail, yet treatments never work. The doctor may not be willing or skilled enough to see the overall pattern of these consultations and sometimes 'break through' to the troubled soul of the patient.

The patient may be freed from this doctor whom they might see as controlling and narrow-minded and the doctor feels relieved knowing that saying, 'Well, you will have to ask the consultant about that' is easier than the further detailed appraisal of the patient's complaint. Some of these patients attend the surgery frequently yet seem to resist any help.

These patients have been called 'black holes' or 'heart sinks' in the medical literature. The descriptions are hostile and punitive, but are a reflection of the way doctors feel. These poor patients seem stuck in a groove, only able to repeat a complaint and find the advice and treatment wanting. Looking at these situations from afar the patient can be seen as desperate for help yet unable to receive it. They are drowning but can't quite accept the lifebuoys thrown to them. In practice, the only way forward is a painful course for a profession programmed to care. The doctor on the boat must call out, 'No one is a good enough swimmer to save you and we can't believe you've stayed afloat for so long.' Slowly the patient starts to swim. If then the doctor on the boat says 'See you're swimming!' the patient will start to sink again. Instead, regular announcements of 'I don't think you'll make it' will encourage the patient to swim. Just being near in the boat is all that's needed.

These black hole/heart sink patients have asked for help from the doctor. Using this paradoxical method the doctor is really saying 'I'm here, I know you are coping with a lot and I'm surprised you want to keep going, many would have given in by now.'

One such patient, an elderly man in his seventies, would come to the surgery to talk about a number of physical complaints. As different doctors tried to help him he would explain that the 'answers' given would not work for one reason or another. The doctors would try harder, but he would always outflank their efforts. He would then return with more complaints and gradually the doctors would feel angry and feel their hearts sink as his name was mentioned.

One of my partners, a family therapist, suggested treating the patient paradoxically. Instead of endlessly trying to get the patient better we should hear the inner voice saying 'I can never get well.' When the patient returned, after listening to the symptoms, he said 'I don't know how you can bear to go on living with all you've got wrong with you.' The effect was dramatic. The patient stood up saying 'Thank you doctor – I'm just going to go on trying for a bit longer.' Over the months he did return occasionally; the observations were repeated such as 'I don't think there's a doctor in the world clever enough to help you.' The reply would come 'Well, at least you tried doctor.' This answer seems harsh and appears to him contrary to the usual patient–doctor behaviour.

This is an effective method that leaves the patient feeling they are understood at last and they are doing the best they can. It will only work in this unusual and particularly difficult patient behaviour.

It is within the scope of family doctors to help with these situations. Referrals for these troubled patients take a large chunk of hospital time and resources. Family doctors are in the best position to help these patients and need to be trained to do so.

Home Visiting

In recent years home visiting has been on the decline. The cause for this is in part because of car ownership and in part because of the improved technology and services available at general practices. This trend will reverse back in the years ahead as the demography of Britain gives increasing numbers of the elderly.

Home visiting will be common in some parts of the country where there is no public transport or difficult local geographic or climatic conditions. Home visiting varies in different countries – particularly high in France and particularly low in the USA.

In Great Britain patients often believe it is their right to demand and obtain a home visit from a doctor. In fact this is not the case. Doctors are expected to make a judgement as to whether a home visit is required and to be prepared to accept the consequences if this judgement is proved wrong. This judgement should depend on knowledge – knowledge not only of the patterns of ill health and of diagnostic skills, but also of the patient, his family and his environment. Disputes over home visiting always occur where there is lack of knowledge. This lack of knowledge may be on both sides.

On face value many requests for visits appear unreasonable:

'My child has a cold, I'd like you to check her.'

But in the next few minutes on the telephone the missing knowledge may be revealed.

Doctor's missing knowledge
Who are this family and what is their experience of ill health? Why do they want me to visit for a cold? What do they understand by a 'cold'? Is this child ill?

Doctor's questions may reveal
  (i)   A new first baby with terrified parents.
  (ii) A family member who has recently been ill or died.
  (iii) A family that does not understand the terms they are using and therefore can give no clear indication of how ill the child is.
  (iv) A family that expects the doctor to call as it is socially inconvenient for parents to come to the surgery or, indeed, inconvenient for the child to be ill at all.
  (v)   A family who believes it is the doctor's duty to call under any circumstances.

Patient's missing knowledge
The patient might be missing:
  (i)   The knowledge of when it is considered reasonable or unreasonable to call the doctor.

(ii) Knowledge of what to do with simple illnesses.

(iii) Knowledge of whether a doctor is there at all and what to do if he/she can't contact one.

(iv) How he/she could act should the child continue to be ill or deteriorate.

(v) Knowledge of the identity of the doctor he/she is talking to, and the doctor's attitude to the phone call.

Patient's questions may reveal

(i) That he/she is dealing with the child's illness correctly and can be left 'in charge'.

(ii) That his/her child is showing no indication of serious illness.

(iii) That he/she does not understand the doctor and does not feel reassured.

(iv) That the doctor is not interested in his/her concern.

These examples are but a glimpse into the complexity of these consultations. In fact, telephone consultation is taught to family doctors in training as it is an important area of clinical skill.

There are many consultations on the telephone in an average family doctor's day – far too many for each to be serviced by a home visit. The family doctors get skilled at picking out the ones that need a home assessment. They do not always get it right.

One afternoon I was called to an elderly lady with a funny turn. She had been in only a week before with giddiness. I had found that this came on when she looked upward or turned her head suddenly. Knowing she had neck arthritis, I was convinced her giddiness was due to the blood being cut off in the neck when she looked upwards. This is a common condition in the elderly and a likely diagnosis.

As her daughter spoke on the phone she explained that 'Mum had had another one of her turns and she put herself to bed.' She mentioned that Mum was very pale and would like me to come now. I knew that this would be the case with one of the turns I diagnosed and reassured her that I would call later if she hadn't recovered.

The daughter rang later on to say her mother seemed to be

sleeping in the darkened bedroom. She wanted me to check her mother anyway before the night. I agreed but remembered thinking it would be a journey wasted. I thought it would probably take a few of these turns before mother and daughter got to know them. They would come to realize that although frightening, patients usually make a swift recovery. On visiting the house the daughter was apologetic and ushered me upstairs. The bedroom was dark and quiet. As I opened the curtains I noticed the bouquet of fresh flowers by the bedside and a deeply comatose patient. It was clear she was unlikely ever to wake up to see her flowers. As I pulled back the bed clothes I noticed the bed was full of purple-black blood. She had been pale from the haemorrhage, not from the 'faintness' as I had thought.

Her daughter was devastated, one moment expecting her mother to wake up, the next realizing she was dying. As usual, the patient's relative was full of self-reproach. How she should have called me sooner, and how she wished she hadn't pulled the curtains. I listened to her and suggested she had done everything a daughter could. We discussed the situation and her daughter didn't want her moved. She died peacefully whilst we were talking. I apologized for not getting there sooner. I expected anger and disappointment, but there was just her self-reproach. I knew angry feelings would come later. I wondered if it would ever be appropriate to talk about how unlikely the haemorrhage had seemed. How I had to take these risks every day, weighing up the needs of a surgery full of people and that of an elderly lady having a turn. Would I be able to discuss what we would have done had I come earlier? Would the elderly woman have wanted to go into hospital and be brought round? Would she have wanted it the way it was?

The incident reminded me that often the patient's relative *senses* that something is wrong. Often that sense cannot be expressed clearly in words. It also reminded me that I should re-check my diagnosis even if I made it only recently. In fact, I was sure of the first diagnosis and later I thought of the pills she took when her arthritis was bad. These pills can irritate the stomach and cause haemorrhages. Perhaps my elderly patient, hearing my diagnosis of arthritis in the neck blocking the blood to her brain decided to take a few more of her arthritis pills. These pills then caused her huge internal haemorrhage. The arthritis was in fact the indirect cause of the final giddy turn.

I would have to judge whether to talk about these things with the daughter in the weeks to come. I knew that I might not get it right then either.

> I was called by a family I know well. They are a happy boisterous family of five living in a large, untidy Victorian house. Although the children were usually grubby and scruffy, I knew they were loved deeply and I had no doubt about the quality of their parenting. Toby, the two-year-old, had been playing with his dad in the living room. He was jumping off one of the chairs and fell into a corner. His dad hauled him out and since then Toby had been crying and holding his arm.
>
> His dad wanted me to come and see Toby. Listening to the story I thought Toby had dislocated one of his forearm bones. This injury is common and easily sorted out. Despite present-day advice to examine any injured child carefully, I decided this could be dealt with over the phone. I was not worried about the possibility of child abuse and this view was supported as Toby's dad made no attempt to hide how the injury occurred. Carefully over the phone I got the father to shake hands with his son, then turn the hand one way, then the next. His father noticed the clunk as the bone resumed its normal position. Toby stopped crying and wanted to romp again with his father.

In this situation the patient wanted a visit and was surprised not to receive it. I was happy not to go as I knew the family well and could trust its judgement. The father was prepared to trust me as he knew that my unwillingness to visit was not just laziness.

All over the country these judgements are made. In the first case I got it wrong. Getting it right might have involved an earlier visit to a dying patient and more support for a worried daughter. In the second case, I got it right, but only because of sufficient knowledge on both sides, patient and doctor.

Finally, a story about home visiting and a battle for who's in charge. In this situation both doctor and patient got it wrong.

I was 'bleeped' by the answering service to say there was an agitated man wanting a doctor for his child, he was making his call from a phone box. I rang back straight away. The consultation didn't start well.

'Hello Mr Tanner, how can I help you?'

'Look, I've just told that woman who takes your messages I want a doctor to come and see my baby.'

'Fine, but I need to ask you some questions first. What do you feel is wrong with her?'

'I don't know, you're the bloody doctor. I told that woman she's not eating and she's throwing up everywhere.'

'How long has this been going on?'

'Look, I'm fed up with this, I'm standing in the road in the middle of the night. If you don't get off your f . . . arse and see my baby now I'll report you.'

'Why are you being so aggressive?'

'I'm not talking any more, just *be here*.'

The phone went dead. What was this all about? I was angry and felt abused. Part of me wanted to refuse to go and to face the music later. We shouldn't have to listen to abuse like this. I then imagined an ill child and a frightened mother and decided to go. When I got to the flat I noticed the door had been smashed and I suspected further violence.

The child by now was asleep. It had vomited and had been hot and her mother explained that they had a niece who had had meningitis. I woke the child and examined her and could find little wrong. I assumed it was a 'viral tummy bug'. I turned to the mother and asked where the baby's father was. He had apparently gone out. I started to tell her of the abusive phone call and she explained he could lose his temper if he was worried about the child. I said it was unacceptable and I would want to speak to him about it. In the next few days I wrote to the man asking to meet him to discuss the incident. As they were relatively new patients I had no further knowledge to go on. No evidence of violence from medical records and the health visitor had only just met them. He made no attempt to contact us or reply to the letter. I was determined not to let it go. In the end, I stated that unless he contacted me in 10 days he would be removed as a patient. He didn't, so he was. As the months passed I reflected on what this battle was about. Was it about an issue of 'who's in charge' or was it just hurt pride on both sides? I realized that I had changed little if he were to call again. I would still have to visit the child and this time there might be a more violent man present who felt worried and rejected.

The situation persists today – the patient has not registered with a new doctor and refuses to discuss the incident at the surgery.

'Who's in Charge' Checklist

1 On leaving the surgery do you know what's wrong with you? Did the doctor seem to agree with your ideas? Do you feel you were understood? Could you have disagreed if the doctor's ideas didn't fit with what you know is wrong?

2 Can you stand up for yourself when it comes to discussing treatment, referrals to hospital, second opinions and home visiting?

3 If not – try and find out why. Is it because:

- You're frightened of upsetting the doctor?
- You feel guilty because others are more ill?
- The doctor has problems of his/her own?
- The doctor won't understand?
- You have always been fearful of authority?

4 Are you happier to leave things as they are, or do you want to change the situation?

5 Changing will mean starting with 'Doctor, I am not sure you understand what I'm saying . . .'

The Medical World

Hospitals: Senses and Feelings

Recently I reminded myself of what it's like to be a patient. Gone was the comfort of the wards and canteen. No longer the banter of difficult 'cases' and dramatic 'incidents'. I was just a patient. I was frightened before my appointment, I was submissive when waiting, and I noticed things I have never noticed before.

First the smell. It isn't just disinfectant, it's a mixture of fumes from X-ray developing and a host of other medical smells. I remembered how, as a junior doctor at last off duty, I would leave the hospital wards and seek fresh air and normal life. It would take a few hours before my sense of smell, dulled by medical smells and dry air, returned. As a patient this is only one sense that is assaulted when coming to hospital.

Second, the noises are alien and disturbing. The bleeping of monitors telling the staff the patient is still alive, the hum of machinery in the background, the urgent footsteps responding to personal pagers, the clank of food trolleys, the whispers of night staff, and the groans of patients in beds.

If this is not enough there is no warning for patients that 'the sights that follow some viewers might find offensive'. As a patient one can't easily switch off. We are likely to see blood on dressings, glimpses of bedbound patients on bedpans and nakedness through curtain chinks. There will be wounds and stitches and patients in pain. There may even be the early morning transfer of the dead body to the false bottomed trolley on its way to the morgue.

This assault on the senses goes unremarked. The staff smile at one another: can't they smell and hear and see? Are they not touched by the pain, the suffering and the distress?

In fact, the staff have been put through a careful programme of desensitization. Their training is an exposure to all of these feelings and more. Human responses are controlled and replaced by measured thought and action. After all, it's no good for the surgeon to be fainting holding the scalpel or for the nurse to be crying whilst dressing the wounds. It is easy to see how this training is needed. It is not clear, however, how this creates a distance between patient and doctor.

Patients, like me, feel outside this world, weak, vulnerable and under assault. Doctors have filtered what they feel and can appear distant and powerful. This distance and power can seep out into their personal lives and stain their relationships. Their friends will admire the things they can't bear to do. The doctor may increasingly be out of touch with the vulnerable inner self. Close relationships often fail.

Patients can help doctors restore some of their balance. They can remind doctors that to wait three hours in pain because of poor internal organization is not good enough. Nor is failing to sit down and really explain without jargon what an operation means. They can also remind doctors that the service is for them so there is little place for patronizing power play and poor communication.

A Doctor

The doctor had been working in the accident and emergency department for two months. Even over those few weeks his confidence had grown: the cut fingers, ill children and broken bones almost felt routine. The nursing staff, kind and supportive at first, now had a growing respect for his new skills. It felt good to be there, in the front line. When a difficult case came along there was help from senior staff. Help especially when new techniques were to be learnt or unusual 'cases' to be seen. The patients were grateful for his magic hands and skills. Then one day an ambulance quietly drove up. The receptionist told the doctor there was a BID (Brought in Dead) to be seen. The doctor said 'Oh I'll do it' as he'd seen many dead bodies by this stage of his training. The ambulance men were getting a cup of tea, a young policeman was sitting on the steps near the ambulance; he was grey and shaking. 'Poor kid' the doctor thought. 'Why don't they prepare policemen for this sort of work?'

The ambulance doors opened to show a stretcher with a red blanket covering a body. Always red blankets, for obvious reasons. As the doctor pulled back the blanket he saw a body in three pieces. The head and torso of this young Black man was in the middle. A shoulder and one arm at the top and the legs at the bottom. He was partially clothed, his eyes were open. The doctor felt his heart pounding and head swimming; he *can* cope with this, it *is* his job. The young policeman explained how he and the ambulance men had picked the bits up off the railway track. No one knew who he was. They would have to search his clothing. They took the stretcher to the Mortuary. With rubber gloves on the doctor picked up the bits of this young man, searched the pockets and then put him in a large plastic bag ready for the Coroner's post-mortem. The policeman grew faint and vomited, the doctor comforted him. Who were this man's relatives? Why had he jumped in front of the train? Where was the train driver and would he ever recover? The word went round the casualty department. A few of the doctor's colleagues wanted to know the details. The horror was hidden by anger and laughter.

Someone had taught the doctor to mend that broken bone, but no one explained how to cope with this. The example of senior colleagues seemed to be cover up, don't show any distress and get on with the job. The doctor got on with the job. That moment is still there inside. What is it about the training, the support, the personality of the doctor that meant real feelings don't get shown? What sort of doctors can manage such cases and not let it change them? Who will ever change the system so that it is different?

A Patient

The patient went to his family doctor because of 'water works' trouble. He had expected it as his father suffered in the same way. After all, at 75 you do expect this. He explained how he had to get up at night twice to pee. How he'd have to rush to the toilet when out for fear of wetting his clothes. The stream was not as good as it was and he tended to dribble urine.

The family doctor suggested a specialist to see if his prostate gland needed a operation. The patient thought this would have to happen. The specialist heard his story, tapped him on the back and said 'We'll sort that out for you. Come into hospital and it will all be explained.' The patient was pleased; it would be nice to get a night's sleep again. In hospital he was cared for by the nurses, checked by a young doctor and asked to sign the consent for operation form. As he was about to sign, the young doctor explained about the operation – the pipe up the penis, the clipping away at the prostate gland and the drainage tube afterwards. The doctor asked if he had any questions. The patient had so many it would have taken all day. The young doctor looked so tired and still had other patients to see. So the patient said 'No'. As he lay there in bed he thought of the questions he might have asked. 'Am I unusual in needing this operation?' 'What can go wrong?' 'Is there a chance I won't be able to hold my water?' 'How painful is it afterwards?' The questions flashed through his mind until the anaesthetist came and examined him and pronounced him fit enough for the operation. The nurse gave him an injection to relax him and then off they went to the operating theatre. The operation did not go well. The surgeon, although experienced with this technique, managed to remove a little too much of the prostate gland. A hole was accidentally made between the prostate and the bowel. This would mean many days in hospital and a risk that he would never be right. He woke up in the ward with a pain in his guts. He looked down to see a pipe coming out his tummy and it was draining red blood. The young doctor said there was a technical hitch but 'Don't worry, we'll put it right – it may take a few more days in hospital.' In fact, it was more than a hitch. The patient developed all sorts of post-operative problems: first, the urine flowed into the bowel and then the stools passed into the urine, all through this little hole. Then the patient got a fever and developed septicaemia and finally developed a clot in the leg that travelled to his lungs and killed him.

The surgeon explained to the patient's family that unfortunately operations do carry a small risk for anybody, and their relative was one of the unlucky ones. The surgeon explained to the junior doctor that according to a world authority on this operation, you can't call yourself experienced unless you've had at least one hole-in-the-bowel patient.

Would this patient have gone forward for this operation if he had known the full risks? How can time be made for fuller explanations and truly informed consent for operations?

The Medical Club

Being in the 'club' means understanding the rules and new members take some time to learn. They must also learn the club language, club dress and club gossip.

Short white coats are the medical students, long white coats the junior doctors; red belts are staff nurses, purple uniforms physiotherapists (or whatever, depending on the hospital).

'I am going to bleed someone' means to take blood; 'I will scope him tomorrow' means to pass a fibreoptic instrument to look inside some part of the anatomy; 'I had a crash call' means someone died and the doctor and nurses were called to try and revive them.

Then, even more abbreviated, are coded signs and symbols for Medical Club Members only:

NG	– New growth (cancer)	GC	– Gonorrhoea
$	– Syphilis	CVA	– Cerebrovascular accident
MI	– Myocardial infarction (heart attack)		(stroke)
BID	– Brought in dead	#	– Fracture

As the new doctors, nurses and paramedical staff join the hospital they are automatically junior members of the 'club'. Once they understand the language and the dress and the coded communication, they will begin to feel like real members. They will begin to hear the club gossip, how one doctor had a disaster in the operating theatre, how someone fainted in casualty or how Dr X is having a relationship with Nurse Y.

So why is the club there? Like most clubs it functions to make members feel they are with a group of people who understand. Club members don't need to explain procedures, actions or feelings. It is understood that some jobs are difficult and upsetting, and there is respect given to members for this. The respect is usually unspoken but it is there. The club is a reminder that when times are hard there are others like you.

Unfortunately, members often forget what it's like not to be included in a club. How does it feel not to be a member of the golf club because you are the wrong type? How does it feel not to be allowed to vote because you are not 18?

The club must be there to keep non-members out and non-members are patients. The fact that everyone is a patient sooner or later is forgotten or blocked out. The patient facing the club will often feel excluded. Who is the member of staff I am talking to? What rank are they? Why do I have to sit here and wait and where have all the staff run off to? Why are only two relatives allowed to visit patients at any one time? Why do the doctors and nurses behave in the way they do?

> The patient was on the ward for the first time. There was relief at getting into hospital after weeks of worry about weight loss and feeling so unwell. On two occasions the nursing staff have taken details of age, address, diet, next of kin, religion: and the young house doctor spent a half-hour asking questions – every bodily function was dissected and discussed. Eventually, the patient was examined from head to toe. Both the questioning and examination had a pattern, and the patient sensed the young doctor was more concerned not to miss part of the pattern than to really consider the answers.
>
> Later, the registrar, a more senior doctor, came to ask a few more searching questions and clarified a few impressions.
>
> Later still the doctors all returned and the young house doctor nervously told the story to his boss, the consultant. He summarized and sorted the pain, the weight loss, in fact the patient's whole life into a medical framework. The patient imagined these people as in a play where everyone had lines except him.
>
> Time passed, the patient experienced other rituals: bedmaking in the morning, the serving of food from large aluminium 'hearses'. At last the patient contacted another 'prisoner' in a nearby bed. 'What are you in for?' They shared bewilderment and concern about what was being acted out on their behalf.
>
> Eventually it's over, all the tests completed and conclusion reached. 'They' seem satisfied but what was it all about? Why did they look so worried when the patient told them one thing, yet looked less worried when some tests came back? Questions were fended, never truly answered. The patient sensed that all *was* well, but only by being in the 'club'. Would he ever really understand what went on?

Who Are the Patients?

Some statistics compiled from the Government's UK Household Survey 1987:

General Practice Consultations in UK: Total

	(millions)
Population in the UK	57.4
Consultations per year	257.0
female	163.0
male	93.0

General Practice Consultations in UK: Age and Sex

Age	Consultations (millions)		
	Female	Male	Total
Under 16	23	22	45
16–44	75	25	100
45–64	31	24	55
64–74	17	11	28
75+	18	10	28

General Practice Consultations in UK: Age group and Location

Age	Location (percentage)	
	Surgery	Home
0–4	83	20
5–15	87	9
16–44	92	6
45–64	87	10
65–74	78	20
75+	51	46

General Practice Consultations in the UK: those (%) who consulted their doctor in the last 14 days

	Age groups for men (M) and women (F)					
	16–44		45–64		65+	
	M	F	M	F	M	F
In work	8	17	9	14	8	9
Unemployed	11	26	14	17	nil	nil
Unable to work (disability/ long-term illnesses)	13	21	27	21	20	18

Who Are the Doctors?

A recent study (Isobel Allen, *Doctors and Their Careers*, Policy Studies Institute, London 1988) interviewed 600 doctors (50 per cent male and 50 per cent female who qualified 1966, 1976, 1981). Some of the results were surprising:

- 50% of students entering medicine are women. (The number qualifying has not changed significantly in the last 10 years, currently at 3600 per year.)
- 65% of females and 50% of males had decided to study medicine by the age of 15.
- Only 7% of male doctors and 16% of women doctors gave wanting to help/work with people as their primary reason for choosing to study medicine.
- The commonest reasons given for studying medicine were 'being good at science subjects' (male 25% and female 19%) or 'good, interesting career' (male 19% and female 15%).
- 42% had a parent, relative or close friend who was in the medical profession, and 25% were influenced in their choice by that person.
- 30% of medical students come from independent schools (a percentage reducing every year).
- 75% of doctors interviewed between the ages of 28 and 45 were married, 19% single and 4% divorced/separated, and only 2% were co-habiting.
- 47% of women doctors were married to male doctors.
- 75% of partners with female doctors were of social class I.

Each year the average family doctor (figures from British Medical Association, Economic Research Unit):

- Prescribes: 14,000 prescriptions costing approx. £100,000
- Gives: 7282 consultations in the surgery
  1285 consultations at home
- Gives: 395 vaccinations
- Provides: 111 patients with family planning
- Treats: 67 temporary residents
- Attends: 38 night visits
- Performs: 47 cervical smears

3 Helpful Hints

Making Sense of a Symptom

Homework

Medical school training for future family doctors instils the importance of approaching each patient's problems in a systematic way. This system starts with a detailed look at the symptom, the circumstances in which it is worse or better, and the duration and intensity of suffering. Then the doctor moves on to direct questions about bodily functions in each system of the body. For example in the heart and blood circulation (cardiovascular system) there would be questions about palpitations, breathlessness, ankle swelling, tolerance of exercise on the flat and on stairs etc. After the systems review, the doctor then moves onto past medical events and family history, social history and each area of the patient's functioning.

This approach is the dragnet approach to the ill patient; it nets a lot of information but only parts of it are useful. It is also time-consuming; a full 'history' and examination will take at least one hour.

In general practice the approach has to be more speargun-like. However, the difficulty is more to be sure that the problem will get 'speared'. Of course, it becomes more likely as the doctor gets to know the patient and vice versa, but also because the patient will return several times if the symptom persists and no adequate explanation is provided.

Current medical training encourages power to stay with the doctors; it is for them to discover, decipher and explain. This approach encourages patient dependence on the medical profession and neglects the healing potential of a patient himself discovering the key to his illness. Clearly, this is not possible with all illnesses. No amount of self analysis will help the patient with appendicitis, but it can sometimes be useful.

A single woman in her fifties would present repeatedly with muscle aches and tiredness. She would describe in detail her pain on rising from bed in the morning and reluctance to face each day. I had examined her on many occasions and found no abnormalities to explain her symptoms. I pressed her to think of the cause but she had noticed no pattern to her suffering. Her only pleasure was a Scottish dancing class and that made no difference to either morning stiffness or exhaustion. I put it to her that such an activity would normally make bodily symptoms worse and maybe the tiredness came from worry or emotional distress. She looked unhappy with this suggestion and asked whether I really believed in her pain. I countered that we all worried and surely she did too. She agreed and said she did get bouts of anxiety but she was unable to specify. I asked her to help to sort it out, she agreed that throughout the following week she would write down every situation that caused anxiety for her.

She returned holding her 'homework'. There were three double-sided A4 sheets covered with writing. Her anxieties spread through every part of her life. She worried that the kettle would break, that the hoover might need emptying. She also worried that she might be disabled and that there would be no one to care for her. She worried she might have multiple sclerosis, tuberculosis or cancer. She worried that she would go mad.

As I read them out, she cried and cried. I sensed I was with someone who felt about five years old rather than a woman of 50. She had made no close relationships but relied on her sister and brother-in-law for support. I discovered they wanted her to move in with them but she feared that she would lose her independence. Over the next few weeks we talked about how to change her situation. She made no mention of her tiredness and morning pain. Eventually she found a sheltered housing unit near to her sister and moved. She wrote later and mentioned her pain and tiredness had gone and how she thought it was because of pollution and the water in London. She made no mention of the work we had done together, asking instead that I should consider London pollution as a cause when other patients came in with her symptoms. I sensed that putting all her worries on paper had somehow made a shift that allowed her to change. I knew that acknowledging this was too difficult for her, but it didn't matter anyway as her pain and exhaustion were gone.

There are other examples of homework used in everyday practice.

A young businessman would always run out of his asthma medicines. He would come to the surgery and get angry and upset if he couldn't have a repeat prescription straight away. The receptionists noticed the pattern and asked me to see him. He denied neglecting his asthma, saying instead that one could never tell when the sprays would run out. I explained that each one had 200 puffs in each canister, and surely he could roughly work out when he would run out if he was using four puffs a day as he said. He became more angry, claiming that doctors didn't know what it was like and anyway some canisters seemed to short change him with fewer than 200 puffs. We were getting nowhere.

I admitted that I wasn't an asthmatic and could see he was in a better position to judge. I asked him to become his own doctor and record his own treatment and its effects. I gave him sufficient inhalers to manage for a couple of months and a machine to record how much 'breath' he had at different times of the day. He suggested he would try different ways of taking his medicine and wanted to try out a new medicine he had read about. We agreed to meet up in two months to review this and he made his appointment. He returned then with detailed charts showing how his asthma had improved on his treatment. He then requested that he should have sufficient medicines in advance to maintain this control. His homework had proved to him that he was the best judge of his asthma and he could control it himself. It unlocked a battle of control between patient and doctor.

Records

There are some symptoms that seem never to fit into the doctor's pattern. They correspond to no known dysfunction of the body and contradict the laws of anatomy:

'When I swallow I can feel my legs tighten and a tingling pain goes down the back of each leg.'

'When I'm constipated I've noticed I get blue rings under each eye.'

These sorts of symptoms cause havoc between doctors and patients. If the doctor says 'I don't understand' or 'I don't know what could cause them' it may feel to the patient that the doctor does not believe these symptoms exist.

It may help to find from the records that these unusual observations have been there for years. Reading the same recorded symptoms from 10 years previously can reassure doctor and patient that although troubling, the symptoms have not progressed to something more dangerous.

One Turkish man came repeatedly about a pain between his anus and his testicles. He was apparently unable to sit for long without moving and had had all his trousers re-made to give him more room. Despite all this his pain continued. As he was a new patient I had little to go on from his records. He explained that his previous doctor had asked him to consult a specialist. He had had many tests and examinations but no one was able to discover the cause.

On examination I too found nothing and suspected that the pain must represent some deep-seated problem. I probed into his sexual and emotional life and found a happy family man with a caring wife and children. He denied any extramarital affairs.

I felt there was something I must be missing but couldn't

imagine what it could be. Just then his records arrived from his previous doctor. Going through these I found pages and pages of doctors' attempts to solve his problem. He had seen numerous specialists and many GPs. He had been to a famous acupuncturist who had written that this symptom is particularly difficult to treat and there had been no improvement over several visits.

I remembered the previous patient with an intractable problem (see p. 103) and the paradoxical manoeuvre. I remarked when he came back that there seemed to be no doctor clever enough to solve his problem. How was he going to face his life ahead with such terrible pain and no relief? To my surprise he smiled broadly and said that he was going to try hard to survive from day to day. I felt he had just been given a medal to pin to his chest with the inscription 'Incurable but struggling on'.

The medical records had shown me that to follow my instinct and refer again would prolong this man's agony. Somehow saying everything's been done lifted his shoulders and his heart.

I was reminded of scenes from epic movies of valour and wounds in battle. I had a sense that modern life devoid of such struggle left this man without a soul. His condition gave him strength and a sense of worth, as if some calling from his ancestors stirred his manhood.

Treatment

What is treatment? In the medical sense I see it as a course of action agreed on between a doctor and a patient in response to a problem. I thought perhaps the word might share its origin with the word treaty: an agreement between people or nations.

In fact, the Latin root of the word 'treatment' is *tractare*, to drag or pull along. Patients who are treatable are pulled along and are docile and manageable.

When we are patients, it is easy to be pulled along by the doctor, but where are we going?

Would we let a stranger tell us when it is safe to cross a road blindfold? How good a friend would we need to have before we trusted him or her to guide us?

We do know roughly how safe it is to cross the road. We also know we can reduce the risk by crossing at the safest place, by looking left and right, and by keeping our ears and eyes open.

When being offered treatment by the doctor, patients should have a similar attitude. They must know the risks they are taking, the consequences of not taking treatment and the likely time-scale of any improvement. In other words, they too must have their wits about them.

Let's look in detail at five areas:

1. Medicines and their side-effects
2. No treatment and its risks
3. Medical fashion
4. Alternative treatment
5. Private care

Medicines and Their Side-effects

Doctors become confident about certain drugs. They are used to prescribing them, and are familiar with their advantages and disadvantages. Most family doctors develop a core of approximately 40 medicines in which they develop trust. The patient may have a deep trust of the doctor and feel, as I described in Chapter 1 (see p. 22), that he or she has negotiated a successful working relationship based on mutual respect and understanding.

In this seemingly perfect scenario both are still at risk. They are at risk because doctors *do* forget and *do* make mistakes; because doctors *do* make assumptions about the patient's attitudes and judgement that are not correct; and because patients *do* feel it is not their business to ask or know about such things as risks of treatment.

How can patients and doctors lessen the risks? First, the decision-making about treatment can be a shared experience. Just as in the section on diagnosis, the choice of treatment is not only decided by the facts of the case but by what is acceptable to the patient.

Until recently part of the difficulty has been caused by lack of information. The largest and most commonly used reference book on medicines' side-effects fails to give a precise indication of the degree of risk. For example:

Penicillin

- Many patients and doctors would use penicillin without too much concern.
- Most will know that allergy can occur and in very rare cases that allergy can kill you.
- Many will know that penicillin can also 'upset your tum' with nausea, vomiting and diarrhoea.
- Most will know of the association of vaginal 'thrush' or candida infection with a recent course of penicillin.
- Few patients and doctors (and I had certainly forgotten before re-reading the reference book) will know that penicillin can cause serious damage to blood cells and kidneys 'once in a blue moon'. But how rare is very rarely, and just what percentage is 'once in a blue moon'? The *patient* may feel *his* percentage is not sufficiently small to take the risk.

More recently, the reference books are starting to quote the precise risks and with the spread of information technology these figures will become more available to both patient and doctor (see Chapter 4). There is no place for the saying 'a little knowledge is a dangerous thing'. No knowledge is even more dangerous and more information can only be safer.

An elderly man came in with swollen, tender knees. He had walked further than usual when visiting his family and was now in considerable pain. I knew him well, and we usually shared gardening tips in addition to the reason for his visit. I knew how much it would mean to him to be deprived of his gardening and suggested an effective course of pills to reduce inflammation in his joints. I warned him they could 'burn' the stomach like aspirin could, and encouraged him to take them morning and evening with food. He asked me if he could take them in the future if he needed to. I explained that there was some evidence that when using the pills the joints got worn more quickly. I was pleased with the interview and thought we had come to an agreement. His knees got better and he continued to take the pills for a few weeks. They had allowed him to sleep without backache and his garden was blooming.

Shortly afterwards I received a call from his daughter to say he was in hospital. He had had a severe stomach haemorrhage and had nearly died. She said the hospital doctors had said it was likely to have happened because of the pills I had prescribed. I felt defensive and worried that I had missed something.

When the patient was out of hospital we discussed the episode. He clearly thought he was dying as he vomited large quantities of fresh blood. I asked him about ulcer symptoms in the past and whether he had got any warning from indigestion. He had had neither and was concerned to know why this had happened. He wanted to know how commonly this drug could cause this problem. I told him that I did not know the precise risks but that I did know they increased with age and the larger quantities of the medicine. Nevertheless, I thought the risk was small enough to keep him gardening. However, he didn't make this decision, I did it for him. I now know the risk of haemorrhage is approximately 1% for the quantities and age of patient involved.

The patient felt that at 0.1% he would have tried the pills but at 1% he would not.

It is not reasonable for the doctor or patient to know all these figures, but it *is* possible and reasonable to make them freely available to encourage informed choices by doctors and patients together.

Medicines and Their Side-effects Checklist

1   Decide whether you do or don't want to know the side-effects of what's been prescribed.

2   Make it clear to the doctor you want to know all about the medicine's side-effects

3   As each medicine has a long list of possible side-

effects, ask the doctor to estimate which are the most
likely problems.

4   Ask the doctor 'If side-effects do occur (e.g. rash,
indigestion etc.) what do I do and how long will they
last?'

5   Ask the doctor, 'Will this medicine need to be taken
repeatedly or should this prescription cure my
problem?'

6   Is it better before or after meals?

7   Will it interfere with my other medicines/foods/alcohol?

8   Do I have to finish the course?

9   Is this medicine really necessary?

No Treatment and Its Risks

Family doctors in training can have great difficulty with this area
of practice. 'What will happen if the patient doesn't take the pills
or follow the advice?' Lacking confidence and experience it feels
as if the responsibility is the young doctor's, and he will be held
accountable when things go wrong. Doctors forget that it is not
their responsiblity to make sure the patient takes the treatment.
It is, however, their responsibility to present the advantages of
treatment together with disadvantages, then to record their
advice in the medical records. Thereafter, assuming the patient is
able to make such judgements, the decision to take the medicine
or not is the patient's. Of course, the patient who refuses treatment for an easily treatable condition causes upset and anger to
doctors. At this stage the doctor needs to stop and consider which
of the patient's beliefs prevent him or her from taking the
doctor's advice; understanding and respect can then follow.

Medical Fashion

George Bernard Shaw's *The Doctor's Dilemma* exposed how
ridiculous doctors can be in pursuing the current vogue in
treatment or advice. The modern-day *Nuciform sac* (a fictitious
fashionable operation) is everywhere:

Then 'You must take iron and vitamins in every pregnancy.'

Now 'We only give iron and vitamins if the tests show you need them.'

Then 'Lowering cholesterol is always good for your health.'

Now 'It seems that lowering it too much can cause other problems.'

Then 'The wonder-drug for arthritis is here.'

Now 'Sorry, it causes ulcers.'

Then 'Eat liver in pregnancy.'

Now 'Don't eat liver in pregnancy.'

No wonder the patient feels confused and doubts medical advice when the passage of time reveals past truths as uncertain. The doctor is just as confused. Tests relied on are now discredited and careful medical advice over years shown to be deleterious to health.

How can patient and doctor avoid medical fashion? I think a suspicion of all new drugs should be a start. Then perhaps reservations when discoveries are found that seem contrary to current belief and practice. This may lead to a conservative profession, cynical and wary about change. Proper cynicism and wariness may seek to control freer spirits in the profession, and encourage eccentricity in other areas. When I look around local practitioners you could not hope to meet a more varied and unusual group of people. Most of them have a particular drum to bang to balance the reserved and neutral stance often needed in the profession.

A High Court judge sought help from his eminent psychiatrist. He wanted a cure for finding himself in seedy dives in the early hours of the morning not knowing where or who he was. The psychiatrist pronounced this as the more normal part of his life, whereas life at the court with control and ceremony uppermost he deemed to be most unhealthy.

Perhaps all professionals need a little area of madness . . .

Alternatives to orthodox treatment

The medical profession is full of wonderful stories and rumours to support its own position. Many doctors delight to tell of alternative treatments being exposed as hocus-pocus and their practitioners as charlatans.

When the Government's pamphlet came through the letter-boxes describing the dangers of Germanium, some orthodox doctors will have had a chuckle. This 'fringe' medicine was one of many recommended by alternative practitioners. It apparently caused a number of symptoms from toxicity.

Then vitamin B6 (Pyridoxine) was found to cause nerve damage when used in high doses and caused dismay in patients who were quite sure they needed the high-dose vitamin supplements.

In one situation the alternatives turned out to be right. A young Nigerian boy was brought in by his mother. He was covered in a red scaly rash which he scratched furiously. She described how his sheets were speckled with blood from intense night-time itching. I thought I knew the best treatments available and was sure we could get him much better. His mother was not worried by the short-term use of steroid creams and understood the need for some sedative anti-itch treatments at night. She diligently followed my advice and his skin barely responded at all. After some weeks I decided it would be best to get the child into hospital for more intensive treatment. The mother politely declined and explained she would be taking her child on a visit to Nigeria. She hoped to see her native doctor who would have a 'natural' cure for eczema. I understood her wish to be home and patronized her by believing that she would get no better treatment there, but at least he might get the benefit of some sunshine. She returned two weeks later and her son's skin was clear. Her native medical man had chosen an ointment made with powdered bark and animal fat. The tub smelt dreadful but the results were remarkable. I was left in no doubt about its efficacy when his eczema returned when the 'ointment' ran out after a few months.

Some time later rumours circulated about a marvellous skin doctor in London's China Town. Apparently families were taking their chilgen there in droves. Many doctors considered this to be the natural but desperate desire to chase any treatment rather than face the reality of long-term complaints like eczema. Shortly afterwards the next rumour suggested that someone had examined the Chinese doctor's 'herbal medicines' and found that they contained steroids. It seemed that orthodox medicine had won the day.

Now, after a recent study in a London hospital the Chinese herbal medicine was found to be effective and to contain no steroids. Indeed, it is now available on an NHS prescription.

Increasingly, the medical world is examining alternative treatments and adopting some. Chiropractic was found to be remarkably effective in a back pain clinic, oil from evening primroses is effective with some skin complaints. The medical profession need not be so nervous of change. It must be prepared to explore new ideas and confront its 'truths'.

Patients are seeking out alternatives, but why are they so attractive? I believe the answer is complex. First, many of the treatments seem to rely on a passive patient and a practitioner with almost magical skills, such as the reflexologist clearing a disturbance in a distant organ. The current belief in orthodox medicine is to reflect responsibility back to the patient and get them to review how their lifestyle could be causing symptoms. This reflection is uncomfortable and the patient may prefer the passive patient role. Secondly, the patient actively seeks these treatments, choosing when to go and choosing to pay for them. They have more control over the arrangements and this is in itself healing.

These factors also apply to orthodox medicine, of course. It is common for patients to be passive and trust the doctor's magic potions or treatments. After all, it surely feels like magic for little white pills to correct a rapid heart beat or put a patient to sleep. It is also true that patients choose to go to the doctor, ask for a specific treatment and they too have paid for the service. Much of the difference may be in the issue of 'Who's in charge' (see p. 90). The choice of alternative treatments may allow the patient to buy the time of the practitioner. This time may be used for an in-depth discussion and description of the complaint. There may be a review of the patient's life and circumstances. The patient has some control over this time and is expecting time to be given to the problem.

With the Health Service family doctor, the patient may be acutely aware of the needs of others and how all have paid for the service. If the doctor appears hurried it may be because of the demands on his time from all his patients. The patient will sense that demanding more time and space may be at the expense of others. The unselfishness of most patients is evident in almost every surgery; the offers of help to elderly disabled, the offers to wait longer while children are seen and offers to come back another time should the doctor be called out on an urgent visit.

The answer may be that the system makes the patient feel like the small cog in the big machine. It always seems there are people in more need. Stressed doctors can easily remind patients of this and increase feelings of guilt and selfishness. For the system to work well it will need patient and doctor to be at their best and frequently neither are.

The alternative therapy bought at the patient's extra expense may also be sought because of the failure of orthodox medicines to bring relief; or, in addition, because of orthodox medicine's failure to make the patient feel special, feel valued or feel understood. But some patients will never feel special, valued and understood.

Here must be the future of family doctoring. By knowing the doctor and knowing the patients, together both can feel special, valued and understood. The relationship is the key. There is little value in staying in a relationship that does not provide these feelings. Patient–doctor relationships are no different from any other.

Private Care

G. B. Shaw suggested that private medicine is open to abuse:

That any sane nation, having observed that you could provide for
the supply of bread by giving bakers a pecuniary interest in baking
for you, should go on to give a surgeon a pecuniary interest in
cutting off your leg, is enough to make one despair of political
humanity. But that is precisely what we have done . . . The process
metaphorically called bleeding the rich man is performed not only
metaphorically but literally every day by surgeons who are quite as
honest as most of us. After all, what harm is there in it? The
surgeon need not take off the rich man's or woman's leg or arm, he
can remove the appendix or the uvula, and leave the patient none
the worse after a fortnight or so in bed, whilst the nurse, the general
practitioner, the apothecary, and the surgeon will be the better.

It is well known that Shaw, as this extract from *The Doctor's
Dilemma* shows, had no time for the medical profession but his
point is well made.

How can patients trust the opinion of a doctor who will
financially gain from a course of treatment prescribed? It is, of
course, down to the professional integrity, honour and con-
science of the doctor concerned.

Although surrounded by kind and conscientious private doctors, I have, from recent personal experience, come to be
suspicious of decision-making where there is a pecuniary
interest involved.

The scene is general practice, founded for all by politician
Aneurin Bevan. The patient comes to the doctor with a 'warty
growth' on the foot or hand. The doctor might suggest to the
patient that these warts are harmless and self-limiting. If,
however, the patient is keen for its removal the doctor might
suggest a pumice stone or some acid paint to apply which could
be bought at the local chemist.

The scene is still general practice, but now the Government
has suggested that family doctors can be paid for each wart
removal. The doctor sees five such warty growths on the patient.
The choice is maintaining the previous advice, full of patient
education and self-sufficiency, or suggesting surgical removal at
approximately £20 each.

As Shaw said, the patient is none the worse. Maintaining

professional values under such pressure is more than a match for most of us.

In health services in other countries doctors are paid for each investigation performed and service given. Patients often feel well cared for in such a set-up, but who is there to prevent unnecessary investigation? The British system favours the payment to follow the patient. So family doctors gain by having more patients on their 'lists'. There is no financial incentive to thoroughly investigate the patient, and the sources are 'rationed' according to attitudes of the doctor concerned. One service seems likely to be expensive and exposes the patient to unnecessary investigations. The other service seems cheap and exposes the patient to minimum satisfactory care.

A recent scenario worried me further.

A woman came in with a fatty lump on her shoulder. Although benign, it annoyed her and became uncomfortable with certain clothes. She wanted it removed. I explained I could remove it for her in the surgery under local anaesthetic later that week. It seemed convenient for the patient, and at £20 from the Government it seemed a fair payment for the work involved. The patient thought about it and then said she would prefer to use her insurance as she had not claimed against it in all her years of cover. I was happy to refer her to a surgeon who was prepared to remove the lump privately. He suggested she came into hospital overnight and duly removed her lump. The result was excellent and the patient delighted.

However, the patient and I were shocked when she received the bill. The surgeon's fee, anaesthetic, hospital bed and analysis came to over £500. The patient felt guilty; she thought she had been indulgent and profligate. I wondered why I was so upset, after all, surely, as Shaw said, the patient was none the worse. I wondered who would really pay for such a system. Perhaps the patient would pay as the annual insurance premiums rose. Perhaps the country would pay eventually as this service was not giving value for money. The jobs involved would surely go when someone finally stopped the profiteering.

United Kingdom Drug Costs

	Total	Per person
1968	£177 million	£3.20
1988	£2527 million (allowing for inflation this figure would be £1106.25 at 1968 prices)	£44.29 (allowing for inflation this figure would be £20 at 1968 prices)

Patient–Doctor Relationship Breakdown

It seems that most patients are happy with their doctors. Recent studies suggest that family doctors are still one of the most trusted professional groups. However, it may give concern to some that the single factor most likely to influence choice of doctor is proximity. This could mean that it is the patient's experience that all doctors are equally excellent or that the patient's expectations of family doctors are so low that any doctor would do.

In general I suspect dissatisfaction is quietly borne by patients, while doctors and the statistics in the studies hide considerable discontent. Fortunately, in many practices the patient may have some degree of choice in which doctor he or she sees. After all, the dissatisfaction may purely be a clash of personalities. Certainly a 'difficult' patient for one doctor may be no problem to another. Similarly, the trusted and knowledgeable doctor to one may appear pompous and ignorant to another. In highly populated areas it will also be possible for the patient to find a new doctor in another practice. In sparsely populated areas there may be little choice but to make the most of a poor relationship.

Increasingly, Vocational Training for General Practice addresses such issues. The post-graduate doctor entering a year of general practice experience will be encouraged to study the patient–doctor relationship, and in particular how this relationship is revealed in the consultation. Hidden discontent will surface in the course of a consultation and cause a 'dysfunctional' interaction (see p. 36) unless addressed directly.

In the previous section on difficulties I have tried to show how discontent should be identified and confronted by doctors and patients. After all, doctors try to encourage patients to look at the causes and feelings associated with a symptom. They may be less willing, however, to encourage patients to look at the causes and feelings associated with their interaction with the doctor. An early discussion about difficulties is likely to improve future contact and may prevent the patient–doctor relationship from breaking down.

Sometimes the 'difficulties' become insurmountable. Disputes over 'who's in charge', 'boundaries' and 'anger' are particularly difficult to contain. Frequently the doctor or the patient feels that the dispute has gone too far. Feelings and pride are too injured to allow re-negotiation. The breakdown is often painful and distressing for both parties. It may follow years of established trust and good communication.

This breakdown may occasionally be over a most serious issue. On the doctor's part this may be so serious as to be regarded as gross negligence or unacceptable conduct. Such behaviour is usually answered in the courts with a legal action taken by the patient against the doctor. Examples of such offences might include sexual harassment, the administration of drugs to hasten death, or being drunk and unable to make professional judgements. If found guilty, the doctor is likely to have his/her 'licence to practise' removed by the General Medical Council.

More commonly the alleged offence is less serious. Nevertheless, the patient may be sufficiently upset to take a complaint to the FHSA (Family Health Services Authority). The FHSA will investigate the complaint and the issue will be resolved by either an informal conciliation service or a formal hearing. The informal approach settles most claims. Both parties would be asked to put their point of view in writing and would then meet together with FHSA staff to discuss the breakdown. Often the patient will have misunderstood the responsibilities of family doctors. Most will only be looking for a formal apology from the doctor. Many complaints will be rejected outright by the FHSA when it is clear that the complainant is mischievous or disturbed.

If the patient or doctor does not want the issue settled

informally then a 'Service Hearing' is called. Such hearings have a legal atmosphere and patients and doctors are allowed to be accompanied by a 'friend'. These may not represent them legally but give advice and support. The patient would be expected to put forward their complaints and the doctor would have to answer them. Alleged complaints might include failure to visit in sufficient time, refusal to refer the patient for a second opinion or refusal to treat a patient. If found guilty, the doctor will be judged in breach of his/her terms and conditions of service. In effect, the doctor will have broken his/her contract to provide care for the patient. The doctor will be fined, or, rather, have future earnings withheld. In addition, the doctor will have the judgement on record and this is considered most serious by the profession. The record of such a service hearing would have to be produced when the doctor applies for future jobs, partnerships and other responsibilities.

So much for the doctors; for the patients the causes of breakdowns are numerous. It is often because of behaviour; perhaps rudeness to staff or threatening behaviour and actual violence. It may be failure to keep to a contract agreed by both parties or failure to turn up at repeated booked appointments. It may also be a breakdown in trust there the patient has sought numerous opinions from a number of doctors and it has become hazardous to proceed with conflicting messages and treatments.

Patient–Doctor Relationship Breakdown Checklist

1   Start by asking yourself what the problem is. Is it a difference in belief or in attitude? Is it a lack of trust or feeling?

2   What is the feeling you have about this problem: anger/ distrust/embarrassment/fear?

3   Use that feeling in your next meeting with the doctor. You might start by saying:
    'I'm angry that you haven't . . .'
    'I distrust the way you . . .'
    'I am embarrassed to say that . . .'
    'I am frightened to discuss this, but . . .'

4   If this seems too much, then a more gentle approach

might be:

'Look Doctor, I feel we're . . .'

'not getting on . . .'

'not understanding each other . . .'

'not going to agree about . . .'

5   After the discussion that follows can you now work with this doctor – can you salvage a good working relationship based on mutual respect for differences?

6   If not, can you change to another doctor in the practice or will it mean moving to another practice?

In the examples that follow the patient–doctor relationship breaks down; sometimes it is repaired, sometimes not. In some the doctor is more at fault; in others, the patient. Each clash of personalities, error or judgement or unresolved emotion is rich in learning for doctors and patients.

An unfit middle-aged woman came to the surgery with chest pain. She described how the pain had come at the end of a busy day. It had spread across her chest and had made her stop for a few minutes. I asked her what she had been doing earlier and she explained how she had lifted some heavy sacks down to the cellar an hour before the pain came on. She knew she had over-extended herself. Her husband insisted she came to the doctor despite her feeling it was all due to the lifting. I carefully examined her and could find nothing wrong. She thought her chest wall was uncomfortable when pressed. I talked to her about the muscles that are attached to each rib and how easy it is to strain them. She felt sure this was the cause.

I explained she could go for investigation at the hospital to make sure it wasn't her heart, but she decided not to take it further unless the pain came back. I suggested she considered regular exercise and took it as a lesson of how important it is to stay active.

Over the next few days she took regular exercise, her ribs ached a little but she expected that. One week later when out with her husband she developed severe chest pains and was admitted to hospital. She spent three days in intensive care. Her husband then transferred her to a private hospital and the specialist apparently told her that my advice of regular exercise and getting fit could have killed her. She had been suffering from heart pain.

Looking back now I allowed the patient's certainty that it was her ribs to blur my clinical judgement. I should perhaps have been more persuasive in recommending hospital investigations with her first attack. I felt guilty and upset. I knew it was useless to try and explain how everyone makes mistakes and how difficult chest pain is to decipher. I had just made an error of judgement and that was that.

The letter I received from the patient was matter of fact. She had decided she wanted to change to another doctor. She could not understand why I hadn't sent her for further tests and she felt she could never trust me in the future.

I decided to visit her at home after her return from hospital. She was initially unwilling but did eventually accept my visit. I apologized and explained how I thought my judgement had been swayed by her hopes that it was nothing serious. She was initially cold and dismissive. I felt cut off. As I spoke her anger erupted and she shouted 'I could have died.' She then started to cry. Her anger then spread. She was angry with the hospital for not explaining what was happening to her. She was especially angry with her family who seemed only to want 'Mum' well again so she could return to her normal duties. She was determined it was going to change and she wasn't going to take on the family's chores ever again. She suspected that years of overwork had brought it on. Finally, she was angry with herself, especially her smoking and obesity.

At the end of this conversation she smiled at me and said 'And I'm still angry with you.' I asked whether she was prepared to give our patient–doctor relationship a second go. She said she would talk it over with her husband and let me know. In fact, I was never told formally but I took her booked appointment two weeks later as a definite yes. And she continues as a patient today and this breakdown in the relationship seems long ago.

On that occasion the central difficulty seemed about a doctor's mistake. Now I see it differently. It was as if both doctor and patient wanted to believe that what they feared would not happen. The patient wanted to hear that it couldn't be her heart, that it had nothing to do with her obesity, smoking and general lack of fitness. The doctor wanted to reassure her that she was right. Both were involved in mutual and self-deception. For the patient chest pain might mean death. For the doctor it was more comfortable to stay in charge and reassure the patient. Failing to confront the real issues and the patient's self-deception was the more comfortable position. The alternative would confront the traditional doctor role, and would mean discomfort for both. It would also mean that the doctor would have to confront his own fitness, future chest pain and eventual death. In visiting the patient at home and facing the 'mistake', the doctor re-established contact with real issues. The patient, faced with a doctor who clearly cared for her, found her anger misplaced. She went some way to putting it where it should be.

This conflict revolved around 'fear of death' and 'who's in charge'. We have talked about these issues since. The patient–doctor relationship has deepened and encouraged the doctor to face other disputes.

A couple would bring their child into the surgery with asthma. This five-year old girl had been repeatedly admitted to hospital with severe asthma attacks. The parents were very attentive and concerned but had difficulty accepting that their daughter needed continuous treatment. Many consultations focused on the parents determination to find 'a cure' for her asthma. It was clear that the idea of asthma ruined their picture of their perfect little girl.

Asthma is a frightening complaint for parents and difficult to adjust to. It is also frightening for doctors and it is difficult to get the balance right when talking to patients. On one hand there is a responsibility to inform of dangers, on the other not to alarm unduly. For successful management there must be a partnership of care and I tried to encourage these parents to monitor and become involved in their daughter's treatment. In spite of this, agreed treatments would be started but then abandoned. I confronted the parents about their inability to follow any treatment through. It emerged that their homeopathic doctor was also prescribing and they didn't like the idea of two conflicting treatments. I agreed and asked them to choose which treatment was going to be tried first. They opted for the homeopathic therapy. I offered to speak to the homeopathic doctor but the parents were unwilling to give me her name. I wondered what this meant and why it was more comfortable for them to keep us apart. I did not press the point as I hoped to continue to work with them should the homeopathic therapy prove ineffective. The hospital admissions continued, their child's asthma remained poorly controlled.

They eventually agreed to try a preventive treatment for their daughter. They seemed to accept that it would take six weeks to truly assess any improvement and they agreed to take no other therapy in that time. We decided to meet every two weeks to monitor progress. I wanted to have frequent contact at this stage, hoping to 'hold' the situation until it was obvious the child was better. I thought at last we were getting somewhere. However, during the second week I received a letter from another doctor describing treatment programmes negotiated at the same time as the discussions with me.

The treatment programmes were similar but the medicines had different names. Had the parents given both treatments to their daughter there would have been some unpleasant and potentially dangerous side-effects.

I decided it was time to call a halt and explained the potentially dangerous situation in a letter to the parents. I also said that I could not continue as the family doctor when so many doctors and treatments were involved. I heard no more until I noticed that the family records had been recalled because they had registered with another doctor.

What had happened? Had the doctor given insufficient space and time for these patients to express their fear and distress about asthma? Had I pushed too hard and too early for them to face the danger and the responsibility? Had I revealed disagreements and disputes in the marriage about decision-making? Perhaps there was a long-standing distrust of doctors dating from childhood. Perhaps also there was a 'simple' personality clash. My decision at the time to withdraw as their family doctor was impulsive and angry. I thought it might be a 'card' that would bring them up sharply to reveal the problem. I felt the child was at risk with these parents. The parents clearly felt their child was more at risk with this doctor. Like so many patients they moved on for one reason or another and I suspect I'll never know what happened.

An elderly woman was dying of heart disease. The difficulty was that she was dying slowly over a couple of years. Each day brought a further restriction of her activities and a reminder of her mortality. She bore this burden quietly and hated to rely on her caring husband. One day she was in agony when constipated, yet too weak to pass the hard motion. I arrived at the house and manually removed the constipated stool. Her husband was relieved as he knew any further effort might have killed her. Her slow decline continued. One morning she called again to say she was in agony once more. She had become constipated despite the laxatives I gave her. She feared for her life as she was so disturbed. I decided that this emergency should wait until I had seen the other patients waiting to be seen in the surgery.

An hour later the call came to say she had collapsed hitting her head and he thought she was dead.

I left the surgery and confirmed she had died. She had been upstairs, going backwards and forwards to the toilet. She was increasingly agitated until she clutched her chest and collapsed on the floor. I lifted her body onto her bed, cleaned the blood from the head wound, closed her eyes and laid her out for her husband to see. He cried and cried. He explained he knew it could happen at any time, and that everything had been done to help her.

Later that day I called to see how he was and found him with the priest. I collected his wife's medicines and said I would call again. In fact I didn't. Time passed quickly and the needs of the ill always seemed to take precedence over the care of the bereaved. I knew he had a supportive family and caring priest and hoped that would be enough. After some months he booked into the surgery. I decided to grasp the bull by the horns and expressed my regret not to have visited him since the death of his wife. He said how surprised he was not to have received any visits since that day. He said his daughter, a general practitioner, prided herself on this personal care, so important to general practice. I explained how impossibly busy it had been and how the recent Government reforms had left even less time for this sort of care. It sounded mean and uncaring. He was hurt and disappointed. He expected the regular visits to his wife would continue for him, especially since he had had so much more trouble with his arthritis since she died. He left unhappy and feeling uncared for. Perhaps his expectations were unrealistic, but I felt even one subsequent visit would have relieved his distress. Over the months that followed he remained distant and disappointed. I have a feeling this is how it will be for the future. The devastating loss of his wife, compounded by the loss of a trusting relationship with his doctor.

It is fortunate that in family doctoring there is more than one chance. I hope in the weeks to come to talk further to this man. Maybe his disappointment is tinged with anger at my failure to come quickly on the second occasion. Perhaps once expressed, he will see that the regular visits he expected are unreasonable. It may be possible then to start talking about his grief and how helpful it might be to talk with others recently bereaved. The local Cruse bereavement service would welcome him and give him the time he needs.

Jane was a drunk. She was well known in the neighbourhood. She wasn't a secretive drinker as many women alcoholics are. She was a 'lurch-across-the-road-narrowly-missing-the-traffic' sort of drinker. She was noisy, abusive and smelly. Despite all this she had something that kept people from hating her. It may have been partly that she reminded them of the music hall clowning drunk and partly that her battered body had actually survived. At the practice we were unusually tolerant, provided she wasn't too noisy. She had to be sober enough to hold a sensible conversation.

For many years this situation continued without a major crisis. However, one day her dog died. She became even more drunk and abusive. One evening she came into the surgery, and after a brief shout at the receptionists she fell asleep in the waiting room. She was there until the last patient had been seen. One of my partners said he would drive her home, and I volunteered to help him. This was a mistake.

Unfortunately, the first disaster was in the car when she was incontinent of urine when strapped into the front seat. Eventually we got her out and managed to take her to her bedsit. We settled her in an armchair and decided to remove any medicines which could have been fatal if combined with that quantity of alcohol. We assessed that she was sufficiently drunk to be oblivious of our burglary, yet safe to be left at home. As we went to leave she noticed the pills were gone and launched herself at us. She felled me with a rugby tackle and struggled to get the pills. I managed to get free and we left with speed. At the practice meeting that followed we considered what action to take. We thought that to have tolerated some of her outrageous behaviour over the years had been to, unwittingly, support her drinking. We decided to take a firmer line. She was warned not to come to the surgery unless sober. If she arrived drunk she would be asked to leave the practice list and to find another doctor. Of course, she was drunk next time and she did have to find another doctor.

Our decision shook her, she thought she would be able to persuade us to change our minds. Eventually she angrily decided to approach another doctor who accepted her, but insisted on stronger guidelines in her behaviour in the surgery. The effect was considerable. She no longer lurched around the neighbourhood and although she still drank to excess managed to behave in a most sociably acceptable manner.

Jane's case reminded me how important it is to have guidelines and rules that apply to all patients. Special arrangements or allowances often end in disaster. Jane did fail to stick to her side of the bargain and the practice failed to make firmer guidelines in the first place.

A young man came in with back pain and wanted pain-killers. He was in agony. He had been abroad travelling in the Far East and had just returned to stay with his elderly mother. He wondered if it was the suitcases he had been carrying. The doctor who saw him knew his mother well and had been aware that he had been away. The doctor left the patient on the couch for comfort and went to get him some pills for the pain from his medical bag. Whilst the doctor was out of the room the young man hopped off the couch, and stole a prescription pad and the doctor's pen. He disappeared out the back door of the surgery. Later that day he was arrested by police as he tried to use a forged prescription to obtain narcotic pain-killers. The doctor concerned wrote to the FHSA requesting the young man's name be removed from the doctor's list of patients.

In situations like these, the event is so serious that trust has been permanently destroyed. Logically it might be better for such patients to stay with the practice where the event is known about and proper arrangements made for the future. In reality the common outcome is removal from the list and forced re-registration at another practice.

Each practice has its limits, it cannot hope to take on and solve all society's problems. The practice team must survive too. The pressure of patients' ill health and the fear and anger associated with it take a toll. If the practice is particularly well organized and supportive, then it may be able to take on difficult problems like the case above.

How to Change Your Doctor Checklist

1 Be sure it's right to change (see checklist p. 135).
2 Find your medical card. (The patient holds this and it is issued by the FHSA. If lost, the practice you are about to register with will apply for a duplicate.)
3 Choose a practice. A list of practices and their services for patients can be obtained from the FHSA or the Post Office.
  Good advice on which practice can sometimes be obtained from neighbours or local chemists.

4   Apply in person, presenting your medical card*,
    or apply by post enclosing your medical card* and a
    letter introducing yourself.
    *The centre section on change of doctor and address
    must be completed.

5   The practice of your choice may have a full complement
    of patients and you may be considered too far away for
    this particular practice.

6   If you disagree with this decision, do try putting in
    writing the special circumstances that make this
    practice suitable for you.

7   If refused, try other practices.

8   If unable to find a suitable practice to register with, write
    to the FHSA with your reasons for requiring particular
    practices in a particular area. They will allocate you to a
    doctor who is then bound to look after you for at least
    six months.

4 Training Future Family Doctors

It takes five years of medical studies to produce a young doctor. This training is lengthy not only to give time to assimilate the facts, but also to practise skills and develop attitudes. This training starts with an almost mechanical analysis of the human condition. How our bodies are made (anatomy), how they function (physiology), how they work at a chemical level (biochemistry). These three areas of study are a natural progression from the biology, chemistry, physics and maths learnt at school.

From the study of normal function, the training then moves on to the study of the abnormal. What happens when illness strikes, how do tissues and cells change? How do organs respond and functions alter? Then there is time for pharmacology, where drug treatments are described and analysed.

This medical curriculum is designed to help young doctors set aside the personal and emotional, and to train them to reflect in a detached and scientific way. By the time they meet patients they will have a background knowledge that would allow a symptom like pain in the abdomen to be viewed on a cellular, hormonal and structural level.

In the final part of their training, the skills of examination are taught: how best to elicit the symptoms from the patient, and how to discover the signs of illness from careful examination. It is left to the behavioural services to try and teach about the patients' feelings and to encourage the young doctors to be sensitive to these.

So future family doctors will have spent five years in this environment, and on qualification face another four years of post-graduate training. These four years will consist of further training in various specialities such as paediatrics, obstetrics, casualty, psychiatry and a full year as a general practice trainee. It is little wonder that trainees dislike the title, implying they are novices when they will be in their ninth or tenth year of training. In the general practice trainee year, the young doctor works closely with an experienced family doctor and learns the skills needed in general practice.

At the beginning of the year, the general practice trainees emerge confident from their medical school and hospital experience. After all, they will have been coping with medical emergencies, doing operations and reviving babies. Within three months, however, their confidence wanes. It will often seem that this lengthy training has not equipped them to deal with the problems and experiences brought by patients to their doctors.

The past training has encouraged them to step back from the patient, analyse, dissect, come to a conclusion and then act. Now they are encouraged to look at the patient as a whole and to try and understand how this person came to feel the way they do. There may also be important influences from their family's social structure to be considered. Many trainees prefer to try and stay in the 'dissecting mode' which is familiar but not appropriate for general practice. General practice relies on the one-to-one relationship as its strength. Does the patient feel the doctor understands her problem? Suddenly the magic of healing is dependent on this interaction between patient and doctor. The trainee doctor can feel exposed not only because he has relied in the past on the hospital team, the structure, the shared responsiblity to protect him, but also because he may be exposed as a *person* for the first time in his training. Suddenly he could be the patient with his own problem to present.

Groups of general practice trainees share the sense of isolation and of being de-skilled in their own roles. Gradually they appreciate the value of their own vulnerability and sensitivity. They discover how being in touch with these feelings helps the patients to feel understood.

In the course of the trainee year these young doctors often have to make a huge adjustment in attitude. They must reach a balance for themselves between models; on the one hand the authoritarian analytical professional, and on the other the 'wounded' self-aware carer.

The former model can stand back and make logical clinical decisions without being personally involved with the suffering and sadness of all he or she sees. On the other hand, this former model may never make enough of a contact with the patient to ever really appreciate the problem. The latter model will make his own feelings available in the interactions with patients. But these feelings, full of sympathy and sensitivity, may blur his or her sound clinical judgement and objectivity.

The development of this balance is the principal goal of general-practice training. It is a balance that can only come after some experiences that touch on deep emotions. It is a reflection of personal maturity. The quest for this balance continues through the family doctor's career.

Carl Jung, the psychologist, describes the presentation of this balance as the 'persona'. Doctors often feel more comfortable with a persona that is closer to the former model. After all, the white coat, the smart clothes, the professional mannered behaviour command the respect of patients and society. It is a drug that is difficult to refuse.

The alternative persona is less addictive; it is personal, private and self-effacing. It seeks to reflect power back to the patient. It is painful and confusing. Just before he died, Jung wrote in his memoirs, 'the more uncertain I have felt about myself, the more there has grown up in me a feeling of kinship with all things'. It is clear that patients are aware of such feelings from doctors and these feelings are healing.

In earlier chapters I have tried to show how much the partnership between patients and doctors determines the quality of care. I believe that the more this partnership is developed, the more rewarding it will be to be a doctor or a patient.

In order to protect this partnership every attempt must be made to encourage doctors and patients to express their feelings, whether in the surgery consultation, in participation groups or in the media. This book has been written in the hope that it will encourage such discussions.

Robin Skynner, the psychiatrist and family therapist, believes that a healthy marriage is one that can tolerate change. I think he is right and it should apply to any relationship, including the patient–doctor relationship.

Future Care

In the next 30 years there are clearly going to be changes to face together. It would seem certain that the patient, through advances in information technology, will have easy access to detailed medical information. This may be available in the home or carried in portable personalized computers. The patient will probably carry their medical records in credit-card-style 'smart cards' which they would bring to the doctor. Information will be shared and the doctor must welcome the challenge of increasingly informed, knowledgeable patients. Although still encouraged by Western medical education, the model of the powerful all-knowing doctor is dying. Its fatal flaw is the tendency to leave the patient powerless. The challenge for the future is in the development of true partnership in health, and encouragement of self-awareness in doctors and patients.

As the patient enters the tunnel of a magnetic resonance imaging scanner, who will have listened to their fears? Who will encourage a discussion about whether to embark on surgery for the tumour that has been revealed? As the infertile couple go for their tenth attempt at 'assisted conception', who will have listened to how they feel about a baby conceived outside their bodies and their fears of deformity?

The more technical and specialized medicine becomes, the greater the need for family doctors. They cannot only be charming, respected pillars of society, nor second-class specialists. They must hope to be what in their hearts they know they are: they are expert listeners and expert talkers; they are in balance; in touch with the patients and their own feelings of how it is to be ill; they are in balance between the advantage of technology and its effects on personality and creativity; they must take risks, be prepared to be wrong and to change constantly. As information technology and economic pressures grow, there will be a temptation not to look at these painful areas listed above. In fact, there will be a greater need to encourage reflection on the important issues of life and death.

Index